Advance Praise for Healing Self-Injury

"Whitlock and Lloyd-Richardson have produced a book that is rigorous, accessible, engaging and full of practical guidance. They lay out a clear and comprehensive foundation to help families understand how self-injury develops, what it means, how it can be treated, and finally—and maybe most important—how young people and families can emerge from this problem with more insight and inner strength, and with stronger connections. I highly recommend this work for anyone seeking a deeper understanding of this complex and vexing phenomenon."

–*Victor Schwartz, MD, Clinical Associate Professor of Psychiatry, NYU School of Medicine, and Chief Medical Officer, The Jed Foundation*

"Drs. Whitlock and Lloyd-Richardson, experts in the field of self-injury, have produced a book that is equal parts evidence-based, empathic, and actionable. Self-injury need not be more frightening and confusing than other problems facing adolescents. I highly recommend this guide to parents seeking to better understand and help with their children's self-injury."

–*E. David Klonsky, PhD, Professor of Psychology, University of British Columbia*

"A must-read for anyone who knows a self-injuring teen! This beautifully written and extraordinarily well-informed guide offers comfort, explanations, and a detailed plan for parents of adolescents suffering from one of today's most troubling and dangerous risky behaviors. Whitlock and Lloyd-Richardson are national experts on self-injury who have translated the science into a remarkably accessible and essential resource!"

–*Mitch Prinstein, PhD, University of North Carolina at Chapel Hill, author of* Popular: Finding Happiness and Success in a World That Cares Too Much About the Wrong Kinds of Relationships

Healing Self-Injury

A Compassionate Guide for Parents and Other Loved Ones

JANIS WHITLOCK

AND

ELIZABETH LLOYD-RICHARDSON

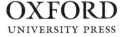

OXFORD
UNIVERSITY PRESS

OXFORD
UNIVERSITY PRESS

Oxford University Press is a department of the University of Oxford. It furthers the University's objective of excellence in research, scholarship, and education by publishing worldwide. Oxford is a registered trade mark of Oxford University Press in the UK and certain other countries.

Published in the United States of America by Oxford University Press
198 Madison Avenue, New York, NY 10016, United States of America.

CIP data is on file at the Library of Congress
ISBN 978–0–19–939160–8

9 8 7 6 5 4
Printed by Sheridan Books, Inc., United States of America

Contents

Preface: Why You and Why Us?

Why Is This Book for You?

If you are the parent of an adolescent or young adult who self-injures or has done so in the past, this book is for you. First and foremost, we want to tell you that despite how helpless you may sometimes feel, *you matter*—a lot. You are a critical part of what happens next. In fact, that's why we wrote this book—and if you are reading it then you may already know this, at least to some degree. It's also likely that you have some questions about what self-injury is, why people do it, and, most importantly, how to help your child, your family, and yourself.

The daily demands of life with children and the need for steadiness and vision, even in the throes of uncertainty and child discontent, is a big, big job—one that can feel very lonely at times and which can leave us feeling like we do not matter at all. In truth, however, you matter in more ways than you probably realize. From us as parents and professionals to you: *You do not need to have it all figured out. Your child did not start self-injuring because you failed. You will not fail your child now if you*

> Your child did not start self-injuring because you failed.

cannot get it all right. You have time. All that really matters at this point is that you are willing to grow, stretch, and learn alongside your child.

It is our goal to help you better understand both your child's behavior *and* your own reactions to it. We hope to increase awareness of patterns that subtly and perhaps not so subtly affect communication between you and your child. And we hope to help you understand the importance of self-compassion and self-care through a time that can be as hard on you as it is on your child.

Why This Book May Not Be for You

For parents of children who are on the autism spectrum or have a developmental disability, you may have picked up this book because you have a child that self-injures in relation to a long-standing disorder. This self-injury is often labeled as *stereotypy* or *self-stimulatory behavior*, and it is repetitive in nature and seen primarily in children with autism spectrum disorders, mental retardation, and developmental disabilities.[16]

In this book, we are primarily referring to *nonsuicidal self-injury* (NSSI) that is not socially visible, but is often chronic, tends to occur in youth with no other clear developmental challenges, and can come and go, sometimes with long periods of silence between episodes. This type of self-injury is commonly viewed by professionals as very different from that which is experienced by individuals with a developmental disability or on the autism spectrum. Stereotyped self-injury is likely observed by parents early in life, perhaps even as early as two to three years of age. These families may have come to some degree of equilibrium as they have learned to work around patterns of behavior and to accommodate family needs in a variety of ways. In these cases, parents typically come to understand self-injury as part of a complex spectrum of behaviors associated with their child's condition, and they would not likely find the information contained within this book to be relevant.

However, a family with a higher functioning teen on the spectrum (formerly known as Asperger's syndrome) who also engages in NSSI may benefit from the material discussed here because it may help to identify ways to develop a deeper connection and to understand what factors trigger your teen's self-injury. Also important, while we rarely think about it in the same way, research shows that caregivers of youth who are experiencing emotional or psychological challenges (such as self-injury, disordered eating, or depression) experience challenges similar to those felt by caregivers of physically or developmentally disabled children or elders.

Why You Matter So Much

While we will examine some of the common family- and parent–child-related issues that may contribute to self-injury, the majority of this book focuses on life after you find out about your child's self-injury. We focus largely on the information and skills likely to assist you in supporting your child's recovery process, as well as yourself and other family members. We focus on this because it has become increasingly clear that parents are critical allies in setting the stage for recovery and thriving. We hope to illustrate how true this is from individual families' stories, as well as from what we know from science and research.

Take, for example, two large studies of young adults and their experience with self-injury. One set of questions specifically asked with whom (e.g., peers, parents, therapists, adult friends, other professionals, etc.) participants had talked about their self-injury and who they thought suspected it. Importantly, it was found that young adults wanted to be able to talk with their parents about self-injury, and they tend to find it helpful when they do. In fact, parents were more likely than anyone else to both initiate a conversation about self-injury and to be regarded by their young adult as the *most helpful* people to talk to about self-injury. In contrast, peers were one of the *least* helpful groups to talk to.

> Young adults want to be able to talk with their parents about self-injury, and they tend to find it helpful when they do.

Another good example of parents making a difference comes from studies of adolescents and young adults in therapy for one or more mental health challenges. While therapy itself is considered helpful, it is much more effective when caretakers are involved and engaged in the process. This is because interactions with parents and caretakers (easy and hard) are part of what forms or describes the "authentic self"—the part of each of us not defined or described by a job or role or by an idea of what we are supposed to be, but which reflects a deeper essence or sense of self. Moreover, it is in families, regardless of the forms they take (traditional or same-sex married, single-parent, divorced, and so on), that children learn that connections to one another matter and that communication between two family members can have effects on other family members and vice versa. These family communications—whether through spoken words, punctuated silence, a roll of the eyes, a disapproving look—clearly impact relations between family members in ways that children observe and learn to interpret regardless of how subtle they are. These exchanges also exert a profound impact on how we see ourselves and, in turn, communicate with others.

By actively participating in the therapy process, parents and caretakers communicate several positive messages to their children, including: "I am willing, I care about you, and I am capable of tolerating the discomfort I am likely to feel at times during this process." The very act of participating, independent of what actually happens in therapy, is a message and influences what happens next.

The communications happening with your teen and within your family are among the primary topics of this book. Readers will come away with tools for understanding how parents' thoughts and beliefs about themselves, their children, and parenting itself strongly shape parent and child reactions to stress and to one another. These personal beliefs can contribute to stress and can set the stage for turmoil if they are not acknowledged and altered. Parents willing to recognize, accept, and heal deep-rooted beliefs and expectations that interfere with their ability to be fully present for their children can expect to see and experience tremendous healing and growth. Parents will also find that taking this step will allow them to be fully present for their child, without feeling the need to fix everything they think is wrong.

Why Us?

For each of us, the path to writing this book was a long and winding road, but one that we each trace to specific moments. We hope that you will find elements of your story here. Although both of us are scientists who study self-injury and related issues, the heart of this book comes from our experience as parents, partners, and friends to other people struggling with this and similar challenges in their families. Between us, we have eight children and step-children, who, at the time we started writing this, ranged in age from 7 to 23. We each have firsthand experience as mothers. And, we are each acutely aware that *life happens in moments, not in big events.* The stories of ourselves, families, and even cultures are crafted through the everyday, often quiet exchange of looks, touch, words, or simple co-existence. We are also both keenly aware of how hard it can be to care for another person and how much we also need support as parents.

Janis

It was deep winter, in 2004, when a dear friend called to update me on her life and family. It had been a rough year, she shared, especially since she had learned recently that her daughter had been cutting herself. In addition to worrying that her daughter was suicidal, she had spent months soul-searching in hopes of understanding how her daughter could have arrived at such a dark place. Seeing the marks that the cuts left on her daughter's arms was viscerally painful for her, and she worried immensely for her daughter's future.

My heart went out to them both, and I was left with a million questions. Having been intrinsically interested in adolescence since I was an adolescent myself, I had given a large chunk of my professional career to understanding and addressing issues related to the adolescent passage. At the age of 25, I had become a "big sister" to a 12-year-old girl I met while working in one of the programs for which I provided sexuality education. I later became a foster parent for her and, through this, became deeply familiar with the way her pain etched itself onto her body—through a persistent eating disorder, nightmares, a seemingly endless array of traumatic memories, deep issues with trust and intimacy, and a profound gratitude for any small kindness an adult showed to her (a rare and sometimes disconcerting orientation for someone of that age). I also, however, witnessed her amazing strength and resilience—a deep well of hope and willingness to trust that her life could be something better, even though she couldn't imagine what or how. It was thanks to her that I began to understand the complex relationship between dark nights of the soul and suffering and the intractable capacity for human hope, recovery, and growth.

However, nothing in my experience with my foster daughter or the vast majority of the young, vulnerable, and troubled high-risk kids I had worked with prepared me for dealing with the issue of self-injury. I was intrigued and also very puzzled after that 2004 call from my friend. When less than a week later another friend confided in me that her child was also a "cutter," my curiosity became too persistent to ignore. Why, I wondered, would a young person growing up in a typical and largely supportive family want to slice, burn, scratch, or otherwise damage his or her body? This curiosity led me on a long and winding road that resulted in research that has dominated the past decade of my professional life and that is chronicled on *The Cornell Research Program on Self-Injury and Recovery* website (www.selfinjury.bctr.cornell.edu); we maintain a wide variety of resources on this website for all who are directly or indirectly affected by self-injury. We will describe this site in more detail in the book's Resources section.

Over the past decade, I have encountered self-injury in my extended family and close friends network, and I've helped one of my children through a hard passage that spanned more than a year and included depression and anxiety, among other things. She, like so many of the young people we talked with for this book, feels emotions very strongly and has struggled to manage them. She has also struggled with a tendency toward negative thinking. This left her less than ideally equipped to meet some of the challenges that life presented. These tendencies, coupled with adolescence itself, culminated in a series of experiences and events that left her on edge.

Over the course of the year that she had periods of strong depression, I experienced first-hand what many of the parents reading this book experience. The need I had to fix her life, to somehow find the combination of ingredients that would resolve all of the perceptions and experiences that hurt her, led me to confront and to ultimately simply co-exist with a fairly chronic sense of powerlessness, vigilance, and hopefulness (during the good moments). It also provided opportunities for growth, expansion, and a sense of surrender that has helped me be a better parent, a better scholar, and a better person.

So, it is my hope that what I share here reflects both my professional experience and my personal experience of parenting a complex child in a complex world.

Elizabeth

Much of my time in graduate school was spent traveling the back roads of Louisiana, heading to various psychiatric hospitals to interview teenagers who had recently been admitted for attempting suicide or who were dangerously close to suicide. I wanted to hear and understand the stories these teens had to share and to learn how their experiences grew to be so different from what I understood to be normal teenage angst. So, in 1996, I began interviewing teens who I thought would serve as a "normal" comparison group to hospitalized youth. I had placed advertisements in local newspapers asking teens to come talk with me in a brief interview in exchange for some small monetary compensation. The teenagers coming to meet with me were normal by all appearances—some came directly from track or cheerleading practice, still in their uniforms; some wore all black, long bangs arching across their faces; some came burdened with heavy backpacks full of that evening's homework.

I was surprised and shocked to learn that many of these teenagers shared dark and troubling stories of emotional pain, a pain they didn't know what to do with, turning it outward and expressing it through cutting, burning, or scraping their own skin.

To be honest, I had never heard of this. My psychology textbooks had taught me that self-injury was rather common among severely mentally disabled individuals as a way to cope with biochemical abnormalities in the brain, or to manage pain, or perhaps to gain social attention. But why would this happen among teens who were of average intelligence, with no disabilities? I could see only the drawbacks of causing injury and pain to the body, but were there hidden benefits to cutting that I was unable to see? *Who* were these teens who were injuring, and *why* were they doing this? These questions were the beginning of my doctoral dissertation, a research project spanning several years, which allowed me a look into hundreds of teenagers' lives.

> Who were these teens who were injuring, and why were they doing this?

More than 400 teens from high schools across the Midwestern and Southern states completed anonymous surveys indicating whether they had ever purposefully injured themselves, what they had done, and why they had done it. The results were shocking. Self-injury did not appear to play favorites. It touched the lives of girls and boys, blacks and whites, poor and wealthy. Roughly one in four teenagers reported harming themselves, with this happening an average of 13 times over the past year. While I was used to working with hospitalized, suicidal teens, I was unprepared to learn that so many teens were experiencing such suffering. Furthermore, teens reported that their self-harm had come to serve a variety of purposes for them, most commonly to stop bad feelings or to feel *something*, even if it was pain.

Over the years I have learned a great deal about who is likely to self-injure and what motivates them to go to these lengths. I have interviewed hundreds of teenagers and young adults about their self-harm, both suicidal and nonsuicidal. I no longer make assumptions about what is or isn't "normal" teenage angst. I appreciate the tremendous work that teenagers have in growing up . . . and I'm not referring to that after-school job they managed to score just down the street. Teens are faced with the prospect of learning how to regulate their time, their ambitions, their relationships, and, perhaps most importantly, their emotions.

My professional work over the past 25 years has shown me that teens use many unhealthy, maladaptive coping strategies to meet their emotional needs. Self-injury can be included along with the usual suspects, such as alcohol and drugs, Internet porn addiction, and eating disorders. While I am aware of all that science has to offer on these topics, I can't help but find myself concerned about my own children's winding path through the teenage years. What will it be like for them? Aside from rolling them up in a thick layer of bubble wrap and duct tape or locking them away in a Rapunzel-like tower, how can I help them develop the skills necessary to navigate these often treacherous waters? They are still young and have a few years before they reach pre-teendom, but, regardless, I have realized that many of the very same strategies and tools that we discuss in this book are useful, too, in laying a healthy foundation of respect, trust, and open communication necessary for the lifelong journey we parents make with our children, no matter what their age. I sincerely hope that you find this book to be as engaging and hopeful as we have felt while writing it.

Acknowledgments

Authors' Note

Throughout these pages, we do our best to tell the personal, often poignant stories of youth and their parents who have taught us so much about nonsuicidal self-injury, growth, and compassion. To protect their privacy, we have changed their names and the details of their lives. We are grateful to every one of these individuals for sharing their stories with us and hope we have served them well with this book and the lessons we have drawn from our work.

Acknowledgments

Much of the science we talk about in this book did not exist even 15 years ago. Self-injury scholars were a rare breed in the early part of the millennia. Early pioneers like Barry Walsh, Wendy Lader, Armando Favazza, and Karen Contario paved the way for a robust crew of dedicated scholars on which all of our current understanding is based: Nancy Heath, David Klonksy, Jennifer Muehlenkamp, Matt Nock, Mitch Prinstein, Kim Gratz, Imke Baetens, Penny Haskings, Stephen Lewis, Paul Plener, Joe Franklin, and the many others who have shined the light of understanding on what we now call nonsuicidal self-injury, this book literally would not have been possible were it not for your work.

Elizabeth and my toils would have been in vain were it not for our two wonderful Oxford editors, Andrea Zekus and Sarah Harrington. Both were essential in helping us shape the book at the outset and then clearly convey the messages we hoped to share in each chapter. Each of their suggestions was exceptionally helpful. Indeed, the whole team at Oxford has been nothing but supportive.

Notes from Janis

Writing a book is so much more work than I ever imagined! I regard the fact that I arrived at the end of this process happy with the book contents and still cherishing my relationship with my coauthor, Elizabeth, as a triumph. Indeed, I strongly suspect that it was precisely because of my co-author, Elizabeth, that I was able to make it to the finish line smiling. From the moment she agreed to undertake this project with me, we made it fun. Long weekends in NYC planning, writing, playing, and simply sharing were strung together with weekly calls to check in on progress as a means of holding ourselves accountable. It worked, though much more slowly than our tidy timeline and division of tasks detailed when we first started out. So, Elizabeth, thank you for being a dear friend and co-conspirator throughout this whole adventure!

Nothing in this book would have been possible without the many colleagues and students who have contributed to building the base of knowledge and understanding on which I leaned while writing this book. In particular, a hearty thanks to Amanda Purington, who so effectively served as the first lab coordinator for the self-injury project and helped to bring forth many of the parent studies on which we drew for this book. Subsequent lab coordinators— Carry Ernhout, Laura Dedmon, and Julia Chapman—have all read chapters, pulled literature, organized parent and child quotes, and generally supported our efforts. Likewise, the many Cornell students who have come through the lab and contributed to the science and translation of science that is discussed here have been an invaluable source of support.

Last, I am deeply indebted to and grateful for my beloved family. Each of you has given me insight, understanding, and a countless number of "ah-ha" moments—all of which ended up in the book in one form or another. It really helped to be raising teens as I was writing. When Elizabeth and I began, mine were just entering the teen years, and, now as we complete it, they are well on their way to adulthood. Aliya, your teenage passages etched an indelible canyon of compassion for all of the youth and parents I wrote for; you were my heart and constant touchstone. Aidan, you fed my steady fire of quiet persistence simply by modeling how it is done with such grace. I so look forward to seeing to what you will bend these traits now that you are entering adulthood! Ravi, you have been instrumental in helping me understand and have deep compassion for the sometimes very narrow passages of minds and hearts in the throes of pain and addiction. I could never have learned what your many years of experience with the layered contours of the human condition have taught me from a book or in a classroom—thank you!

Notes from Elizabeth

Words cannot express the admiration I have for my co-author and dear friend, Janis. I am grateful to have such a compassionate, grounded friend with a brilliant, curious intellect. We didn't exactly know what this adventure would bring for us when we started, but we jumped in with both feet, and I'm glad it was with you that I've traveled down this path! I've enjoyed our weekly conference calls, writing meetings, walks in Central Park, and wide-ranging conversations over tasty vegetarian dinners at Blossom. You are a special and strong woman and make the world a better place. I look forward to exploring what trouble we can get into in the future!

I am grateful for my students over the years, who have listened to me sort out the things that I struggled to get out of my head and onto the pages of this book—Briana Paulo, Joana Goncalves, Andrea Avecilla, Angela Darosh, Lucia Andrade, Angela Dibenedetto, Patrick Geuder, and Olivia Covino, among others. I have grown from knowing and collaborating with each of you, and I hope you find joy and satisfaction in your professional careers ahead.

Special thanks go to my husband, Tom, who read drafts of various sections of this book without complaint and always offered helpful comments. More than that, you have been supportive of this project from the start, and I appreciate more than you can know your unwavering support and encouragement in my abilities to write for families that I have the greatest respect for. I am grateful also for my own parents—Iris, Paul, Donna, and Leon—who have offered the type of support, encouragement, and communication that everyone should experience from their family and friends. And Mom, your home-cooked meals that you periodically provided helped me to write for just a little longer some days, knowing that my family would have a healthy, tasty meal to enjoy! My sweet and salty children—Max, Summer, and Daicey—were young when I started this project. I still think they may be inclined to believe that I was "just watching Netflix" all of those times that I declared, "Mom's busy now, I'm trying to get a section of the book written." Well, here is your proof! I hope we can always keep talking and laughing with one another, allowing us to get through the good and not so good times. Thank you all for your patience as I persisted with working on a project that hopefully offers useful information, guidance, and solutions to families that struggle with helping a child who self-injures.

Why This Book and Why Now?

THIS BOOK RESULTS FROM YEARS OF IN-DEPTH CONVERSATIONS, surveys, and interviews with youth and parents of youth who self-injure. It also comes from a growing number of studies, from the United States and from abroad, that persistently show that parents play a particularly powerful role in the recovery process. All of these sources portray parents who care, parents who worry, and parents who are willing and able to stick by their children through the sometimes very rocky terrain that can mark this passage.

Our studies also reveal how parents are affected—parents whose physical, social, emotional, spiritual, and overall mental health and well-being can be profoundly impacted by living with children who injure their bodies, the bodies that their parents helped to create and nurture. It can be difficult for parents to watch their child suffer, particularly when that suffering is brought about at the child's own hand. And, in cases where parents have contributed to their children's suffering, the guilt and shame can be crippling.

If you are reading this book, then you have already taken the first step. You are clearly a parent who cares; a parent who should know that you are not alone; and that, when your child begins the recovery process, you are likely to play a critical role as supporter, cheerleader, and role model for how to manage the ups and downs of a rocky road to recovery.

Preview of What Is to Come

We are just two of a growing number of scholars whose curiosity about self-injury led them to investigate it in the early part of the new millennium. We are now part of a caring cadre of researchers and clinicians in the United States, Europe, Australia, Canada, China, and a number of other places around the world exploring self-injury and its relationship to other mental health challenges, emotion regulation, cognition, family structure, how it may spread from one individual to another, and a variety of other topics that will comprise the science reported in this book.

The goal of this book is to help you understand where your child's self-injury comes from; why he or she does it; and how to help your child identify, build, and use skills that will assist him or her in recovering from and growing beyond self-injury. We also hope to help parents understand that there are rich opportunities for personal and familial growth as a result of the process of recovering from self-injury. Indeed, many young people and their families can and do find healing, closer relationships, and deeper levels of communication and authentic living as a result of navigating this challenge.

> We hope to help parents understand that there are rich opportunities for personal and familial growth as a result of the process of recovering from self-injury.

In service to these goals, this book is divided into four sections. The first gives an overview of self-injury, what it is, how common it is, and what we know about those who self-injure. Included is consideration of the factors that lead to self-injury and how inner thoughts and feelings can interact with outside factors, like family, peers, and school, to affect development of and recovery from self-injury. We discuss in detail the role of the family and how your understanding of these factors is critical to your ability to aid in your child's successful recovery and growth.

The second section is devoted to recovery, treatment, and review of the skills that individuals who injure typically need in order to overcome self-injury impulses and behaviors. We talk about common types of treatment and how these are used to develop the key skill areas and strategies needed for recovery. We expect that knowing about these issues will help you identify what might be contributing to your child's self-injury. In this section, we will also help you assess your child's stage of readiness to change. Understanding the basic recovery process is often key to treatment and recovery work. We'll also help you understand how to reframe your experience from disorder to discovery, including new ways of thinking about what progress and recovery mean.

The third section shows you how you can be your child's partner in the healing process. Based on information you've gathered, we recommend activities, strategies, and other ways to help support the recovery process. We focus on developing skills to improve mindfulness, regulate emotions, and manage negative thoughts. We also address the limits of what you can realistically do and the profound importance of taking care of yourself in the process.

The fourth section is devoted to dealing with the "practical matters" common in families with a child who self-injures—issues related to the nuts and bolts of talking about self-injury productively; negotiating specific issues associated with self-injury such as safety contracts, power struggles, and access to self-injury implements; and developing strategies for obtaining support from people around you. While you may consider jumping right to this section to get started, we hope that you'll hang with us through the first few sections as we walk you through information we know is critical to understanding and effectively using these practical skills.

The knowledge, skills, and tools included throughout this book are based on our years of clinical and research work in this area; interviews with individuals who self-injure, as well as with parents and therapists; and our understanding of current research on these issues. We hope that we can provide you with answers to your many questions about self-injury and with useful strategies for how to best help your child. Where we think it will help, we include comments from some of the many parents and youth we have worked or spoken with as part of our research. While the names attributed to each comment are pseudonyms, the ages and actual comments have not been modified other than to omit obscuring words such as "um" and "uh."

Preparing for the Activities and Reflection Exercises in this Book

In almost every chapter you will find activities, reflection exercises, and/or worksheets that are intended to help you understand and apply the concepts and skills that we review. In preparation, we suggest that you dedicate a journal for recording your activity responses, thoughts, impressions, or takeaways. This may be a journal you already have, one that you purchased for this process, or something that you keep electronically. Don't worry, we don't expect you're going to completely fill it, although you might! Mostly it's an opportunity to keep all of your work, reflections, and epiphanies in one place as you move through the book. It can be helpful to look it over when you're done or even as you go along.

Reflection Activity 1

Reflection Activity 1: Intention Setting

In preparation for the effort that you will put into learning from this book, it is helpful to take a few minutes to consider what you want from it. The Parenting Intention Worksheet located at the end of this Introduction is designed to help you reflect on this and to set your *parenting intentions.*

As you probably know, an "intention" is an act of deciding on a goal or purpose. It is like deciding on a general place you want to go and then finding the North Star in the night sky by which to navigate in that general direction. While the terrain you will cross may be unknown, your sense of where you want to go and why you want to go there is generally constant. What you may not know about the word "intention" is that it also refers to *the act or fact of healing,* or *the healing process,* in medical lexicons. How appropriate is that? Like planning for a trip or family vacation, there is still so much to learn about your destination, what you might encounter along the way, and how you might best prepare. Similarly, the process of healing begins with an intention. This intention doesn't specify the how; it can only describe the desire and the general location of one's desire. In other words, an intention can inspire and can direct our attention, focus, and purpose—but the how and actual experience of the journey is usually unknown.

> An intention can inspire and can direct our attention, focus, and purpose—but the how and actual experience of the journey is usually unknown.

Take a few minutes now to complete the Parenting Intention Worksheet with regard to parenting your child through this time. Why did you pick up this book? What are you hoping you'll get from it? Most importantly, as a parent, what do you hope to communicate to or encourage, support, or engender in your child right now? It will be especially interesting to revisit these thoughts when you're done with this book, or along the way when things get confusing or frustrating.

Parenting Intention Worksheet

1. What values do you want to teach your child? This might include, for example, valuing respect, the importance of friendships, respect for authority, a strong sense of integrity, a deep connection to family. In other words, what do you hope your child will value and hold dear as he or she moves into adulthood and beyond? Write down two or three that are important to you.

_____

_____

_____

_____

_____

_____

2. What skills do you hope that your child will have mastered or be on her way to mastering by the time she reaches adulthood? This might include, for example, the capacity for deep honesty, the ability to work really hard even when she wants to quit, or being able to manage money well. In other words, what do you hope your child will be able to do well as he or she moves into adulthood and beyond? Write down two or three that are important to you.

_____

_____

_____

_____

_____

_____

3. Write down two or three examples of how you know that you already model these values and skills for your child. Record one set for values and one set for skills (e.g., if you value respect, how do you demonstrate respect to your child? If you value emotional regulation and balance, how do you demonstrate these to your child?). Please provide three brief examples. Be as specific as possible.

   1. Value: _____

      How do you demonstrate this value? _____

      _____

   2. Value: _____

      How do you demonstrate this value? _____

      _____

   3. Value: _____

      How do you demonstrate this value? _____

      _____

4. Can you think of one or two examples where your behavior might not be in line with your intentions? Most of us have areas of misalignment. These are places where we value something, but that isn't really the way we live or we don't really communicate that. For example, we may value eating healthy fully but demonstrate that we can't live without our one Diet Coke every day. Or, we may say we value being honest but notice that we hold back a lot of our true feelings and thoughts. Can you find a few places where you are not in good alignment with any of the parenting intentions you have identified?

   _____

   _____

   _____

   _____

   _____

   _____

5. What are 1–3 ways you want to show care and love for *your child* in the coming year?

_____

_____

_____

_____

_____

_____

6. What are 1–3 ways you want to show care and love *to yourself* in the coming year?

_____

_____

_____

_____

_____

_____

7. What are 1–3 things you would like to learn from this book?

_____

_____

_____

_____

_____

_____

Section 1
Nonsuicidal Self-Injury (NSSI) Background and Basics

The Basics of Self-Injury

At thirteen, Tracy is the epitome of a junior high schooler—worried about fitting in, growing up, and reconciling a somewhat turbulent past with the promise of future independence. One night, after a particularly volatile exchange with her mother followed by a disappointing experience with her best friend, Tracy's agitation is palpable. At the pinnacle of her distress, Tracy makes her way to the bathroom and reaches for a pair of small scissors stored in the vanity. Although a typical piece of bathroom paraphernalia, for Tracy the scissors perform a particular and unusual function. Sinking to the floor, blades in hand, she slides the sharp edge across her wrist—lightly enough to avoid serious injury, but deep enough to cause blood to well up as it slowly passes over the delicate skin. On her wrist lie the tell-tale signs of other, similar moments. After one long cut, she lets the blades fall drunkenly from her hand, as she covers her wounds with her shirt sleeve—already stained with dried blood. Tracy is now very calm; her anxiety soothed by a sort of drug she has not had to buy, steal, or imbibe.

—From the movie *Thirteen*[1]

TRACY'S STORY, DEPICTED IN THE FILM *THIRTEEN*, IS RELEVANT for many reasons. One of these is that her tendency to cut when she feels stress is reflective of what some have called an "epidemic" among youth.[2] Nonsuicidal self-injury (NSSI), the deliberate destruction of body tissue without suicidal intent, is increasingly common in adolescent and young adult populations. Although most often associated with the term "cutting," self-injury includes other self-harming behaviors such as intentional carving of the skin, scratching, burning, embedding objects in skin, or swallowing toxic substances.

As we will talk about in more detail in the next chapters, studies of the origins of self-injury suggest that it stems from a complex array of factors but almost always involves challenges with managing emotions and negative thoughts. Parents play a particularly powerful role in helping children and youth learn about emotions and about effective strategies for coping with them. So, it is not surprising that the parent–child relationship is important in both the development and the continuation of teen self-injury.

What Is Self-Injury?

Throughout this book, when we discuss NSSI (or the shortened form, "self-injury"), we use the definition provided by the International Society for the Study of Self-Injury (ISSS). It defines self-injury as the "deliberate destruction of body tissue without suicidal intent and for purposes not socially sanctioned."[3] The "socially sanctioned purposes" component of the definition refers to body alterations pursued for aesthetic purposes such as tattooing and piercing. Although these may appear self-injurious, they are often undertaken for aesthetic or ritualistic purposes; they are relatively common practices in today's society and are so excluded from the formal definition.

In our experience, self-injury can be cyclical—meaning that it can happen frequently for some period of time (days, weeks, or months) and then stop, sometimes for very long periods of time—maybe even years. It is not uncommon for people to engage in periods of high and low frequency with sometimes long periods of no injury in between, only to begin again. This cyclical pattern can leave parents uncertain about whether the behavior has stopped for good.

In general, it is important to know that the primary marker of NSSI is not the specific form it takes, but the intent: people who self-injure inflict wounds on their bodies in order to alter their emotional states. Although the specific behaviors employed as part of self-injury are easy to confuse with suicide attempts, NSSI is, by definition, largely devoid of suicidal intent, and, paradoxically, most often signals a strong desire to live and to feel better. This caveat is particularly important and powerful: self-injury typically emerges from a desire to feel better, not to end one's life. This impulse, the desire to feel better, is critical; it can be worked with and built on. If you need something to focus on when times are hard, remember this critical point.

> Self-injury typically emerges from a desire to feel better, not to end one's life.

While the intent is not to kill oneself, some forms of self-injury can lead to serious medical consequences, including death. The relationship between self-injury and suicide is a complex one and worthy of further discussion. We will talk more about this relationship a little further into this chapter.

Science Spotlight: DSM-5 and the Diagnostic Criteria for NSSI

In the newest edition of the American Psychiatric Association's *Diagnostic and Statistical Manual of Mental Disorders* (DSM-5),[4,5] NSSI is designated as a diagnosis "in need of more research." That is not to say that experts crafting the DSM do not believe that it exists, but instead that more research is needed to better understand who self-injures, how self-injury should be defined, and what psychological symptoms occur alongside self-injury. This is a significant improvement over previous editions of the DSM that mentioned NSSI only when referring to the criteria for diagnosis of borderline personality disorder, a persistent psychological condition involving a pattern of unstable interpersonal relationships, emotions, and self-image. The inclusion of NSSI in the DSM-5 as a disorder requiring further research indicates that self-injury can be viewed as a psychological condition in its own right and allows mental health professionals the use of a common language for discussing self-injury among their clients.

Information regarding the severity, frequency, and the purposes that self-injury serves for your teen will be important for a psychologist or psychiatrist to consider when determining whether he or she meets the clinical diagnostic criteria for NSSI. Importantly, a thorough clinical assessment is necessary in order to evaluate for any other medical or psychological conditions that may be contributing to a person's behavior. The proposed NSSI diagnostic criteria include five or more days of intentional self-injury without suicidal intent in the past year with the goal of seeking relief from a negative feeling or cognitive state, expressing or resolving a challenge with one or more other people, or to induce a positive state. The diagnostic criteria also require that the behavior be associated with at least one of these: difficulty with relationships, negative feelings and thoughts (e.g., depression, anxiety), planning the act beforehand, or ruminating on NSSI. Behaviors undertaken for aesthetic purposes or as part of a subgroup, such as body piercing and/or tattooing, are not part of the proposed diagnosis. Nail biting and scab picking are also excluded.

How Common Is Self-Injury?

Perhaps it will help for you to know that you are far from alone. Despite how isolating self-injury can be for families, it is increasingly common. Rates of self-injury vary rather widely depending on the research study. It is generally estimated that 12–37.2% of all adolescents and young adults have self-injured at some point in their lives. In a recent meta-analysis (a review and integration of all studies to date) across the world, researchers calculated an international lifetime prevalence of 17.2% for adolescents, 13% for young adults, and 5.5% for adults.[6] Among people who possess other identified psychiatric conditions, such as those in clinical treatment for depression, anxiety, or borderline personality disorder, 65% of adolescents report having engaged in self-injury. In short, self-injury is far more common than most people know.

When Does It Start?

Most studies show an average age of initiation between 11 and 15 years, but a sizable number of young people report starting earlier or later in adolescence or early adulthood. About 6–7% of adolescents and young adults report having self-injured within the last 6 months. For many teens, self-injury is a phase that lasts from 1 to 5 years and then stops. For about 20% of those who start as an adolescent, self-injury is the beginning of a behavioral habit that becomes increasingly difficult to stop.[7] This is one of the reasons that early detection and intervention is important.

Who Self-Injures?

There is no typical self-injurer "profile." Self-injury is widespread and appears in a wide variety of young people—high achievers, shy kids, boys and girls, popular kids, athletes, kids with abuse or trauma history, and every other group found in most schools and communities. Because many of those who self-injure function well in life, it is easy for self-injury to go undetected for long periods of time.

There are minimal differences in the rates of self-injury by race, ethnicity, or socioeconomic status. While some large studies find that white youth are a little more likely to self-injure than those from other groups, the differences are very small. Moreover, studies of self-injury across various countries of the world reveal prevalence rates that are very similar to those in the United States. Self-injury exists in every country studied around the world.[8]

You might be surprised to learn that self-injury is not unique to adolescents. It's estimated that 4–8% of adults have self-injured, and a large study in Australia found that children as young as 10 and adults as old as 84 had self-injured in the month before taking the survey.[9] In fact, the same survey identified people in their 60s who had injured for the first time in their lives—so, clearly, this is a behavior that is not specific to youth.

In short, people who self-injure can be found in families just like yours or ours. Self-injury is not a commentary on who a person is or where she or he comes from, nor does it reveal anything about one's quality of family life or parenting. In fact, there are few things we can say for sure about all youth who self-injure or about their families. Some things that people who self-injure seem to have in common are that they feel emotions very strongly (even if this leads to a perception of deep emotional numbness), are likely to be highly critical of themselves (and often of others), and may direct a lot of negative emotions toward themselves. Indeed, self-criticism has been shown to be one of the best predictors of persistent self-injury. Nevertheless, the path to self-injury can be variable, which means it's nearly impossible to predict who will self-injure and who will not.

> The path to self-injury can be variable, which means it's nearly impossible to predict who will self-injure and who will not.

Does this mean that where young people live, who they interact with, and what they experience in childhood doesn't matter? Not at all: there are trends worth talking about. But, keep in mind that trends rely on averages, and it is rare to find any particular person or family that represents the "average" across any phenomenon. Nevertheless, statistics are often useful in helping us get a sense of a particular phenomenon or behavior and the patterns we find, particularly if they keep showing up in a variety of studies.

Is There a Link Between Gender and Self-Injury?

Self-injury is commonly associated with females in the popular press and in our culture. However, most studies suggest that there is little or no difference in the rates of self-injury between females and males, and this seems to be the case in the United States and in other countries. In studies that do find some difference, it's relatively small (females are about 1.5 times more likely to injure than males, so the ratio is about 35% male and 65% female). In sum, despite popular conceptions of how self-injury varies by gender, there are few if any differences in self-injury rates among females and males.[10]

What, then, might account for the rather popular cultural idea that self-injury is a "girl" thing? Perhaps it's that the presentation of self-injury in males and females can be pretty different. While it is clear that there are a significant number of males engaging in high-severity self-injury (about 30% of all high-severity cases), self-injury among males can "look" quite different from that among females. In the following list we outline a few differences in the typical self-injury of females versus males found in one of our studies.[11] In general, you will notice a pattern in which self-injury begins for females as a means of soliciting attention but may be maintained largely by a desire to manage uncomfortable feelings. Self-injury among males, on the other hand, often looks like common aggression (hitting and punching) and can be easily written off as "masculine behavior." Females are more likely than males to:

- Report more self-injury incidents and more commonly use cutting as a form of self-injury
- Damage their arms, wrists, thighs, and calves or ankles
- Start injuring because they were upset, wanted someone to notice, or wanted to shock or hurt someone
- Use self-injury to regulate emotion or as a form of self-control
- Have difficulty controlling their urge to self-injure
- Injure in private, going through phases marked by high and low NSSI activity
- Have friends who self-injure
- Seek medical assistance for severe injuries
- Believe that self-injury is a problem in their lives
- Attend therapy for any reason (not just for self-injury)

In contrast, males are more likely than females to:

- Bang or punch objects with the intent of hurting themselves
- Injure their hands
- Start injuring because they were angry at someone or because they were drunk or high
- Injure themselves more severely than expected and be under the influence of drugs or alcohol when this occurred
- Use self-injury to get a rush or surge of energy

- Sometimes injure themselves in the presence of others or let others cause injuries

To summarize, the research to date suggests that, for females, chronic self-injury may begin for a variety of reasons (such as learning from peers or social media about how it helps to manage emotions or perhaps as a means of soliciting attention) but may be continued largely by a desire to manage feelings. While the majority of girls describe injuring only in private, fewer boys report this as a private act, and some boys (12%) injure in the presence of others as part of social rituals (e.g., dares or as part of proving masculinity). The notable absence of males in media representations of self-injury largely reflects the fact that a lot of male self-injury looks like typical aggression and can be easily written off as a masculine behavior. Male self-injury is also much less visible in the mental health arena since males are two times less likely to be seen in therapy for any reason *and* are less likely to disclose that they self-injure to their therapist. Males are also less likely than females to regard self-injury as a problem, and it is often much easier for them to hide self-injury—at least for a while.

Is There a Link Between Sexual Orientation and Self-Injury?

The one demographic area in which there are clear trends in self-injury is sexual orientation. In fact, sexual orientation is the only demographic characteristic to be consistently linked to self-injury. Sexual orientation refers to whom someone is sexually attracted to or aroused by, and it is commonly identified as straight/heterosexual, bisexual, gay/lesbian/homosexual, or questioning.

Rates of self-injury among gay and lesbian youth are slightly higher than in those of straight youth. However, differences in self-injury rates are particularly pronounced when comparing straight young people to bisexual or questioning youth. Males of various sexual orientations do not appear to differ dramatically in their likelihood of self-injuring. However, rates of self-injury among females identifying as bisexual or questioning are often near 50%. Moreover, sexual orientation is highly predictive of risk for self-injury, with heterosexual females at lowest risk and bisexual females at highest risk.[12]

Why would this be? As with the link between suicide and sexual orientation, the reason for elevated risk may not be sexual orientation, per se, but instead risk factors that come as a result of being a sexual minority, such as heightened stigma or confusion about how one fits into broader society. Females have a long history of using their bodies as a billboard for self-expression. We can see this historically through fashion, jewelry, makeup, and, more recently, with piercings and tattoos. That women would also express confusion, stress, and distress over their sexual identity through bodily alterations and markings is consistent with such historical trends.

Overall, the research linking self-injury and sexual orientation suggests that it may be fruitful for parents and other adults involved with self-injurious youth to be aware of the young person's experience, challenges, and perceptions related to sexual identity. If self-injury is an expression of distress and/or confusion rooted in sexual identity or orientation experiences, then it may be most helpful for parents to acknowledge those beliefs and experiences that may have led to a child's distress, self-injury, and the need for self-expression. Since sexual identity, orientation, and other perceptions or behaviors linked to sexuality can pose a lot of discomfort for families, simply being willing to engage in candid conversation with an open heart and mind can be immensely helpful and allow for growth in your relationship. If you suspect that your child struggles in these areas and has not been able to be honest with you, we encourage you to find support in starting the conversation and keeping the doors open. You will find that this serves many goals and is very likely to reduce self-injury.

> It may be fruitful for parents and other adults involved with self-injurious youth to be aware of the young person's experience, challenges, and perceptions related to sexual identity.

How People Self-Injure

The most common forms of self-injury reported by adolescents, young adults, and adults include scratching, cutting; punching or banging objects with the conscious intention of injuring; punching or banging oneself; biting, ripping, or tearing the skin; carving on oneself; and burning oneself. There are, however, a wide array of

Box 1.1 Forms of Nonsuicidal Self-Injury

NSSI can include a variety of behaviors. These include, but are not limited to:

- Intentionally carving words or symbols on the skin
- Cutting the skin
- Subdermal tissue scratching
- Burning (e.g., cigarettes) or branding oneself
- Friction burn (e.g., rubbing an eraser across skin)
- Banging or punching objects or oneself with the intention of hurting oneself
- Hitting self (e.g., with hammer)
- Biting self
- Pulling out hair
- Picking at or interfering with wound healing
- Head-banging (more often seen with autism or severe mental retardation)
- Multiple piercings or tattooing*
- Embedding objects under the skin
- Ripping or tearing skin
- Rubbing sharp objects, such as glass, into the skin
- Breaking bones
- Amputation

*May be socially sanctioned or approved but also may be a type of self-injury, especially if pain or stress relief is part of the reason they do it.

forms that people use to injure—not all of which are listed here (see Box 1.1).

"Cutting," or use of some sharp implement like a knife or razor blade, is the form that people most often think of when they hear the word "self-injury" and is one of the dominant forms that people use. However, this can be misleading as many young people may under-report the breadth, depth, and form(s) of their self-injury to parents and other individuals close to them.

I remember the first time I cut myself was with a tin can, which was what was available when I got pissed at that time. It wasn't a plan or decision. It wasn't like "I'm going to use this knife and cut myself," it was whatever was available. That first cut was stupid. I didn't do it out of anger but out of a bet with someone. I said I'd rather cut my-self than blah blah blah. And the guy was like, do it then! And I did it. That is how it started.

—*Siang, age 20, on his first self-injury episode*

For example, although most parents assume that youth use a single method to injure, the majority (between 50% and 70%) of self-injurious individuals report using multiple methods and injuring multiple places on the body (arms, wrists, hands, thighs, stomach, and calves or ankles are the most common, but no body part is ex-empt). Parents are extremely likely to have inaccurate information on the type and number of forms used by their children. Indeed, one of our current studies comparing youth and parent reports found that parents consistently underestimated the number and forms used by their children, as well as the occurrence of self-injury episodes. More than half of the youth surveyed reported using two or more forms of self-injury, while only one of the parents surveyed was aware of this. More than half of the youth reported using other forms in-cluding burning, hitting/bruising, and severe scratching. Notably, many parents were under the impression that their teens had stopped injuring. While only about a third (36%) of the adolescents reported that they had stopped self-injury, a full two-thirds (67%) of the parents believed that their children had stopped injuring.

Because of the variation in how young people injure themselves, the extent of body damage incurred as a result of the practice also varies widely. Unfortunately, it is rather common for more injury to be caused than was intended. In one study, more than a third of respondents said that they should have been seen by a medical profes-sional for one or more of their injuries; only 6.5% reported actually seeking medical attention.[13] Similar findings have been reported in a large study examining self-harm among secondary school students in the United Kingdom, in which 12.6% of adolescents reporting any self-harming behavior reported seeking medical attention.[14]

Stories such as this are common:

One of the last times I did it was triggered by a horrible fear of aban-donment. I grabbed a knife, which I had used before for this, that I actually kept in my book bag, pulled it out, and just kind of went "slash—slash—slash—slash" several times across my stomach. I was so revved up from everything, I did it much harder and deeper than I ever had before. I remember I cut across my belly button. I had a cut that started one side and kind of jumped over my belly button and went over to the other side, and it was just incredible. So it was bleeding pretty bad and opened pretty bad so I knew I needed to do something. I felt as though I couldn't call anybody else because I didn't want to get in trouble for that. So, I called my brother. I think he just immediately understood my desire to not have anybody know. So, he just bandaged me up and told me everything would be fine. . . . I just remember sitting there thinking, "I can't believe I did this, this is horrible. People are going to find out." No one ever found out.

—*Melanie, 25, on her worst self-injury episode*

In summary, it is common for people who self-injure to be using multiple forms of injury, to be doing it in multiple places on their bodies, and to be at risk of unintended severe injury. It is also common for this diversity of practice and experience to be minimized or not reported at all to parents and others who are directly involved in the care of teens who self-injure.

Other General Patterns to Know About

Those who self-injure chronically often have rituals or "private practices" of some form or another that allow for a high degree of control. For example, we know that self-injury is prompted largely by the experience of negative emotions. For some, this can mean that an episode of self-injury is unplanned and happens in response to an unexpected negative event or emotion. Others may plan their injury episodes in advance, deciding when, where, and what tools they will use hours or even days ahead of time. Some people have a strong preference for a particular room, time of day, set of tools, and/or frame of mind. Some people describe keeping a bag that contains their supplies needed for self-injuring always ready for quick and easy access. Parts of the body affected can also have meaning, sometimes of symbolic importance. Most common are arms, wrists, hands, thighs, stomach, and calves/ankles. Wounds and scars may be well-hidden or visible depending on desire for social recognition. Wounds on the face or genital region are almost always an indicator of severe trauma and other significant psychiatric conditions.

Although the majority of individuals who practice self-injury report it as a private practice for managing their own emotional reactions and for which they are not consciously seeking attention, some individuals use self-injury as a form of social bonding. Indeed, in one study of self-injury in high schools, about 25% of the nurses, counselors, and social workers who responded said that they knew of students who self-injured as part of group membership, some on school grounds.[15] In these cases, the regular "practice" of self-injury manages emotions and also is likely linked to what is happening socially and/or what one hopes to communicate to others, often parents or peers.

It is common for someone who self-injures to go through periods of high and low activity with weeks, months, even years in between episodes. This can be confusing for loved ones because it may look and feel like the self-injury behavior is over for good when that is not actually the case. We generally consider people well on their way to self-injury recovery when it has been a year since the last injury, and we consider them stable in recovery when it has been more than 3 years since the last self-injury and when the person feels confident that he or she won't do it again.

> It is common for someone who self-injures to go through periods of high and low activity with weeks, months, even years in between episodes.

Self-injury can become so routine that it looks and feels like an addiction. While there is evidence that injurers have no need to injure if things are going well, it is also true that some people, like Sara (quoted here), start to notice that even small negative events can trigger an urge. While we typically reserve use of the term "addiction" in reference to a substance that is taken into the body, comments about the addictive nature of self-injury are very common among individuals who injure regularly:

> Now, it's like anything will trigger it. And before it hit addiction stage it was specific to the situation with my girlfriend. Later anything would trigger it. Being told I did something wrong was a big trigger because then I would think "oh I'm a bad person, I need to punish

myself so no one else has to." Or still having a fight with my dad was a biggie. My dad came for Christmas and that's the last time I hurt myself lately.

—*Sara, age 19*

What Other Mental Health Challenges Go Along with Self-Injury?

As you may have learned first-hand, it is common for people who self-injure to also be suffering from other mental health or behavioral challenges. For example, it is not uncommon to see disordered eating, depression, anxiety, borderline personality disorder, posttraumatic stress disorder (PTSD), and sometimes substance use disorders in conjunction with self-injury. In fact, it is rare for individuals who self-injure to *not* struggle with other mental health challenges. Among one sample of adolescents admitted to a psychiatric hospital and who had engaged in self-injury in the past year, 87% met criteria for at least one mental health diagnosis.[16]

Science Spotlight: What's the Connection Between NSSI and Borderline Personality Disorder?

The most recent edition of the *Diagnostic and Statistical Manual of Mental Disorders* (DSM-5),[5] classifies NSSI as a condition for further study. Prior to this, NSSI was included in earlier versions of the DSM only as a symptom of borderline personality disorder (BPD). You may have heard about BPD, sometimes called "borderline." Those with a diagnosis of BPD often experience intense and unstable emotions that can shift quickly. They have difficulties calming down after an emotional outburst, and they engage in impulsive behaviors: substance abuse, risky sex, binge eating, and self-injury, are common. For these reasons, those with BPD are likely to use self-injury to regulate their emotions, relieve tension, reduce unpleasant feelings, or regain control over a dissociative state.[17] According to psychologist Matthew Nock and colleagues, 52% of a sample of hospitalized adolescents who had engaged in self-injury in the previous year met criteria for BPD.[18]

The experience of BPD and self-injury is connected by several key factors. Individuals experiencing either of these conditions often have difficulties with identifying how they are feeling, they have trouble regulating their emotions and impulses, and they experience greater distrust of others in their social relationships.[19] According to a review of the literature, individuals who engage in NSSI and also have a diagnosis of BPD are more likely to engage in more frequent and more severe methods of self-injury.[20] They are also more likely to have been diagnosed with other DSM conditions, particularly anxiety disorders, severe depression, and suicidal ideation. Those with BPD have described their emotional state before self-injury as full of "strong tension or pressure," empty, lonely, or depressed/sad, with these emotions often decreasing after a self-injury episode, at least for a brief time.[21]

Despite a strong relationship between self-injury and BPD, not all those with a diagnosis of BPD engage in self-injury, nor do all those who self-injure meet criteria for BPD.[22] For this reason, should your loved one receive a BPD diagnosis because of a history of self-injury, you should feel comfortable asking the mental health professional what led him or her to diagnose BPD. A diagnosis should not be made as a knee-jerk reaction to hearing about a history of self-injury. Diagnosis should really be about all of the symptoms the individual is experiencing, namely: impairments in self-functioning (e.g., instable goals, identity, values) and interpersonal functioning (e.g., difficulty recognizing feelings/needs of others or intense, unstable relationships), as well as negative affect, impulsivity, risk-taking, and anger/irritability.[5] It is also important to note that BPD is one of the most misunderstood and stigmatizing conditions (patients with BPD can be labeled as "treatment resistant," "manipulative," and "drama queens") by the general public as well as by mental health clinicians. Because of this, it is important that an *accurate* diagnosis is received that is based on symptoms and not just the name given to classify them.[23]

While youth who self-injure may also struggle with other impulsive risk behaviors, like drug or alcohol use or risky sex, this overlap is less common than one might assume. Notably, in one study of 30 adolescents and young adults asked to provide real-time data on self-injury and suicidal thoughts and actions over a 2-week period, participants reported thinking about self-injury in conjunction with drugs or alcohol 15–20% of the time but actually engaging in self-injury in conjunction with drugs and/or alcohol only 3% of the time.[24]

For parents of youth dealing with multiple mental health challenges, many of which may be happening simultaneously, life can feel overwhelming. Although effective treatment may vary based on the particular constellation of factors your child struggles with, sorting through the various issues at work and responding in ways that are both productive and feasible take time and patience. We will talk about common therapeutic approaches for treating multiple mental health challenge cases in Chapter 7.

What's the Relationship Between NSSI and Suicide?

That self-injury and suicide behaviors are related is well-documented at this point. The particular nature of the relationship, however, is complex. Because NSSI and suicide-related behaviors can *look* so similar, it can be very difficult to tell the difference between them. In general, the most important distinction is the *intention and medical lethality of the behavior*. It is important to know that NSSI is virtually always used to *feel better rather than to end one's life*. Indeed, some people who self-injure are clear that it helps them to *avoid* suicide. NSSI and suicide differ[25] in multiple ways, including:

Expressed intent: The expressed intent of NSSI is almost always to feel better, whereas for suicide it is to end feeling (and, hence, life) altogether.

The method used: Methods for NSSI typically cause damage to the surface of the body only; suicide-related behaviors are much more lethal. Notably, it is very uncommon for individuals who practice NSSI and who are also suicidal to identify the same methods for each purpose.

Level of damage and lethality: NSSI is often carried out using methods designed to damage the body but not to lethally injure the body badly enough to require treatment or to end life. Suicide attempts are typically more lethal than standard NSSI methods.

Frequency: NSSI is often used regularly or off and on to manage stress and other emotions; suicide-related behaviors are much more rare.

Level of psychological pain: The level of psychological distress experienced in NSSI is often significantly lower than that which gives rise to suicidal thoughts and behaviors. Moreover, NSSI tends to reduce arousal for many of those who use it and, for many individuals who have considered suicide, is used as a way to avoid attempting suicide.

Presence of cognitive constriction: Cognitive constriction is black-and-white thinking—seeing things as all or nothing, good or bad, one way or the other. It allows for very little ambiguity. Individuals who are suicidal often experience high cognitive constriction; the intensity of cognitive constriction is less severe in individuals who use NSSI as a coping mechanism.

Aftermath: The aftermath of NSSI and suicide can be strikingly different. Although unintentional death does occur with NSSI, it is not common. The aftermath of a typical NSSI incident is short-term improvement in sense of well-being and functioning. The aftermath of a suicide-related gesture or attempt is precisely the opposite.

Despite differences and intention, suicidal thoughts and behaviors and NSSI do share common risk factors such as high emotional sensitivity; history of trauma, abuse, or chronic stress; very strong emotion or lack of emotion; tendency to suppress emotions coupled with few effective mechanisms for dealing with emotional stress; feelings of isolation (this can be invisible in people who seem to have many friends/connections); and history of alcohol or substance abuse. *Because of this, it is important for you to know that youth who self-injure are also at increased risk for suicidality.* Our work[26] shows that about 65% of youth who self-injure will also be suicidal at some point (though many will not go beyond having suicidal thoughts). For many, NSSI is used alone or in combination with other behaviors as a way to keep emotional distress or disconnectedness at a manageable level. Although suicidal thoughts and behaviors can occur before self-injury is used, in most cases, suicidal thoughts and behaviors coincide with or come after self-injury starts. It is also important to note that only 36% of adult injurers in the United States reported having ever felt suicidal while engaging in self-injury, meaning that the majority of injurers have never felt suicidal while engaging in self-injury.[27]

Although self-injury does not *cause* suicide, the other important thing to know about the relationship between self-injury and suicide is that the very act of engaging in NSSI reduces inhibition to suicidal behavior if someone becomes suicidal. In other words, having "practiced" injuring the body repeatedly makes it easier to actually injure the body with suicidal intent. Other risk factors we have seen in our studies[28] that place someone at greater risk of moving from self-injury to suicide include:

- Greater family conflict and poor relationship with parents
- More than 20 lifetime NSSI incidents
- Psychological distress in the past 30 days
- A history of emotional or sexual trauma
- Greater feelings of hopelessness
- Identifying self-hatred, wanting to feel something, practicing or avoiding suicide as reasons for self-injury
- High impulsivity and engagement in risky behaviors
- Substance use
- A diagnosis of major depressive disorder (MDD) or PTSD

These risk factors may be present individually or in clusters. The more of these your child has, the higher his or her risk is of at least having suicidal thoughts (this is called "suicidal ideation"). What is important for you to know is that one of the most powerful *protective factors* against moving from self-injury to suicide is a feeling of connectedness to parents. The very fact that you are reading this book says that you are a parent who cares deeply and who is willing to do whatever you can to connect to your child, so please do take this to heart. Indeed, the consistency with which parents show up in our studies as important sources of support for their children is one of the reasons we wrote this book!

Activity

Reflection Activity

Based on your reading of this chapter material, we encourage you to reflect here on what you have learned and how this information may relate to your own life and personal situation.

1. What is the most surprising detail that you learned from this chapter? Why?

2. Think about your own child who self-injures. What are your concerns for him or her right now?

The Family Experience of Self-Injury

Tina's daughter, Sophie, was what she called a "cutter." Sophie had started cutting at age 14 in response, her mom thought, to a rising tide of stress related to school, peers, family, and inner pressure that drove her to be a bit more tightly wound than other kids. The family had moved a couple of times when Sophie was young, and her father suffered from an illness that left him unavailable at times, but overall Sophie's childhood had been pretty typical—certainly not one her parents thought would lead to her cutting herself. In her social and school life, Sophie masked her inner discomfort reasonably well. Although Sophie had become somewhat more withdrawn and moody over the past year, it was not until Tina received a call from Sophie's school that she became aware of her daughter's self-injury problem.

—Family Interview summary

When You Care for Someone Who Self-Injures

Sophie's case highlights a common theme among those who self-injure: she lives with and is loved by family members who are at a loss about how to address a behavior that looks and feels like a suicide attempt. It's a behavior that most parents do not understand and feel helpless to prevent. What many parents do not understand is that, despite the fact that it often *looks* like a suicide attempt, self-injury among most teens is best understood as a way of *coping with stressful emotions and thoughts*. Indeed, self-injury is often an unhealthy response to a very normal and healthy desire to feel better. This last part is important to highlight since the desire to feel better offers something to build on in the recovery process.

Taking the optimistic view, however, can be difficult when you see fresh wounds or scars that may never fully disappear, or when someone you care about seems to be suffering in ways that are hard to understand or to remedy. It can be even more difficult when the self-injury behavior(s) are not all that's going on, when someone you love is showing signs of depression, anxiety, disordered eating, posttraumatic stress, or borderline personality disorder. In these cases, the self-injury itself seems to be just one of a constellation of symptoms whose origin can feel elusive and difficult to treat. How do you react to a person who goes through phases of cutting his or her body but who seems fine otherwise? Or, conversely, who seems to have so many other challenges that it is hard to know where to start? How do you know when to react and when to stay quiet? How do you know what to do when you react? How do you know when the self-injury has really stopped versus when it's on hiatus? And, how do you take care of yourself and the rest of your family members in the midst of the emotional and physical turmoil that seems to come along with the behavior?

These are just some of the questions that parents, caretakers, and others who care for individuals who self-injure confront. In many cases, self-injury behavior is just the tip of the iceberg. And, since the size and shape of the iceberg below can be very different from person to person, finding useful treatment and knowing

> In many cases, self-injury behavior is just the tip of the iceberg.

how to effectively navigate life with someone who self-injures can be difficult for families. Before we get to this though, let's start with addressing some of the basics.

Living with Someone Who Self-Injures

Not all self-injury is the same. Like depression or anxiety or other mental illness diagnoses, self-injury is a behavior that can exist alone or as part of a wide variety of other conditions. This not only makes treatment complex, it means that families with self-injurious members may face different sets of challenges.

There are, however, a few relative constants. The experience of knowing that someone you love is physically hurting themselves and may hurt themselves lethally someday is one of these constants. As a result of this, many family members or loved ones live with some level of stress, fear, or a constant worry that it will start again. Hypervigilance can also cause imbalances in the way attention is directed in families, sometimes resulting in more attention for the child who is struggling, to the detriment of other family members, such as siblings or even a spouse/partner. And, there is a certain level of secondary stress that parents or other caretakers of self-injurious youth experience as a result of the added burden of logistical support, emotional worry, and existential concerns.

In cases where self-injury has been long-standing, families may have come to some degree of equilibrium as they have learned to work around patterns of behavior and to accommodate family needs in a variety of ways. In cases where self-injury starts later in life, usually in or near adolescence, and/or in which it is combined with other symptoms, such as depression, anxiety, or disordered eating, families can find themselves confused about what is happening and how to best respond in ways that support their self-injurious child *and* other family members.

When You First Find Out

It seems like every time I climb a mountain and come to a solution, there's just another part—you know it's like the pioneers crossing

> the Rockies, right? And every time you get over one mountain, you
> look and there's another huge mountain in your way. So that's
> kinda how I felt, it was like, "oh jeez, here we go again."
>
> —Tom, parent of teen with self-injury history

In some cases, parents of young people who injure learn about their child's self-injury through some dramatic experience. For instance, in Sasha's case, her parents found out when she was admitted to the Emergency Room because of what her camp counselors thought was a suicide attempt (she insisted it was not). Steve found out about his daughter's self-injury through her school—an unexpected call he received in the middle of the day. Receiving a call from a school counselor is one of the most common ways to find out about self-injury, although what happens from there is variable. Most often, parents are asked to come in and talk with one or more school administrators. While these conversations range from really unhelpful to really helpful, they almost always come as a surprise and tend to generate anxiety for parents.

In many instances, however, you will have noticed signs of something before you found out about the self-injury. There may have been clues such as depression, anxiety, suicidal thoughts and/or behaviors, or other clearly identified psychological challenges. Your child may have started spending more and more time disconnected or alone. He may have retreated to his room and started spending hours online or otherwise away from the rest of his life. Old friends may have drifted away. Sometimes a parent has a notion that something is not quite right but cannot put a finger on it, such as in Tonya's case:

> "Well, you know," I said, "Have you been drinking?" And she said no,
> and I said, "I'm so glad to hear that because I know that was hard for
> you," and she said, "Yeah, but I've been doing other stupid things."
> I asked what and she said cutting. And I was floored.
>
> —Tonya, parent of teen who self-injures

Many parents, however, find out about their child's self-injury slowly. Pieces of a puzzle come together as signs and symptoms build up, such as wounds or drops of blood in the bathroom, and a parent takes the step of initiating a conversation. In most cases, self-injury is one of several signs that a child is struggling with mental and emotional health challenges. The fact that self-injury commonly co-occurs with other mental health challenges can leave parents feeling like self-injury is just one more (or the first of many) reminders that a child is failing to thrive.

> In most cases, self-injury is one of several signs that a child is struggling with mental and emotional health challenges.

The feelings that arise for parents in the wake of finding out are almost always very intense and fraught with worry or guilt, at least for a little while. In our work, we notice that many parents blame themselves to some degree and tend to see their children's behaviors as a reflection on themselves and how they may have failed as parents.

Is This My Fault?

I couldn't stop shaking. I remember wondering how I missed it, you know. I guess [I was] kind of upset with myself . . . how did my kid get to this point and why didn't I know what was going on? When I see the marks, it makes me feel worse about myself, like I didn't do a good job, like I made mistakes.

—Tina, on finding out about Sophie's self-injury

This has to be the single most common concern that parents report. More than 75% of parents surveyed in a recent study said they felt guilty and worried that they somehow contributed to the onset or maintenance of their child's self-injury.[1] Chantelle's reaction to finding out about her daughter's self-injury is similar:

I am confused and feel broken after having provided her with everything a mother is supposed to provide to her children. I've been a great mother. I listen, I give them what they need, I support their interests, I laugh with them, play with them, travel with them. I don't understand how to help her through this, and it feels like the biggest curve ball of my life. I fear for her life.

—Chantelle, parent of a teen who self-injures

The role that families and parents play in behaviors like self-injury is complicated. We will explain what research tells us about the relationship of families to self-injury, but first we want you to know this: no matter how your child arrived at this place and no matter what you may wish you had done differently, what matters most is what you do now.

Parents are particularly important to their child's recovery process because parents model strategies for expressing and managing strong emotions, whether they are aware of this or not. Additionally, parents' thoughts and beliefs about themselves, their children, and parenting itself strongly shape parent and child responses to stress and to each other. These beliefs can set the stage for turmoil but can also allow for deep healing and growth if parents are able and willing to become aware of deep-rooted beliefs and expectations that may be interfering with their own ability to support their children.

Links Between Families and Self-Injury

Our family life has not been ideal. I have been through a hard divorce, and his mother and I fought a lot at the beginning. Neither of us were very warm people emotionally. Sam just kinda got lost in it all. We have all learned how to be more there for each other from this.

—Tom, parent of teen with self-injury history

While parents do not *cause* complex behaviors like nonsuicidal self-injury (NSSI), things that happen in families and/or during childhood can play a role in the development and/or continuation of self-injury. We know, for example, that for some youth self-injury is a result of sexual, physical, and emotional abuse. This is because abuse of any sort is strongly linked to development of a sense of self-hatred or self-directed negative emotions, low ability to identify and verbalize emotions, emotional volatility and a blurry sense of self–other boundaries. These limitations tend to lead to reliance on harmful strategies, such as self-injury, to cope with intense feelings of inner conflict. However, many teenagers who self-injure do not report ever experiencing abuse or, for that matter, other significant family stressors.

Parenting Style

Decades of research provide ample support for the benefits of using positive "authoritative" styles in rearing children.[2] While the effects of this style vary, it is generally agreed that more supportive and less harsh forms of parenting tend to be most beneficial. Authoritative parents are warm and supportive of their children, but also provide consistent and firm rules and management. They are neither neglectful, excessively permissive, or highly controlling and critical. This type of parenting style has been associated with many positive outcomes. It's also associated with less likelihood of experiencing poor academic performance, substance abuse, or teen pregnancy. As you might expect, research also shows that authoritative parenting is linked to low self-injury risk. Parents who are emotionally distant and overly controlling, with excessive rules or criticism, tend to have teens with increased self-injury risk. Parents able to walk the fine line between providing firm and sound expectations and behavioral consequences while also maintaining compassion and connection (even if not all at once!) are in the best position to help buffer their adolescents' ups and downs and to make recovery from major life challenges—like self-injury—easier. It is important to note that each of us knows a number of parents who have adeptly and consistently practiced authoritative parenting styles and whose children still struggled with self-injury, so having a child who self-injures is not always an indicator of less than ideal parenting styles.

Family Dynamics

Current research on self-injury and families tends to focus largely on family dynamics as a possible contributor to the onset or continuation of self-injury. Not surprisingly, many of these studies do find a link between family dysfunction and onset and/or maintenance of self-injury.[3] Many individuals who self-injure tend to feel emotion very strongly and tend to report more negative thoughts than do people who don't self-injure. This can lead to them feeling more isolated and contribute to the experience of strong negative emotions, which can lead to self-injuring. Is this cycle due to *real* parental issues, with a need to exert more control over a teen than is healthy? Or perhaps it is the teen's *perception* that interactions with parents are more negative than they might really be? Or maybe the issue is that parents are less likely to use an authoritative parenting style with teens who self-injure, out of fear of giving them too much freedom because it may lead to more self-injury?

Whether self-injury is a result of parenting practices, parent–child attachment, or familial events, or whether it reflects a temperamental predisposition that affects the way an individual *perceives* interactions with others, is not clear (in all likelihood, it is some combination of both). What is clear is that *perceived alienation, criticism, and disconnectedness from others*, particularly parents, play a major role in perpetuating self-injury.

> Perceived alienation, criticism, and disconnectedness from others, particularly parents, play a major role in perpetuating self-injury.

Transgenerational Patterns of Stress

In all likelihood, biology and environment interact to influence the family dynamics of self-injury. For example, we consistently see that parents with children who self-injure are more likely to report current or past mental health challenges of their own, such as depression. This link suggests a genetic predisposition to mental health issues. Parent mental health challenges may also affect how a parent interacts with a child and/or teen. Lydia's mom, for example, was depressed and anxious often when Lydia was a child. Despite wanting to protect Lydia and her brother from threat, she inadvertently modeled fearful living to Lydia. This was compounded by Lydia's early childhood sexual abuse by an uncle:

> My mom is really anxious—different than me. It's not that she doesn't feel safe for herself. She doesn't feel safe for me or my brother. Because she really hates herself and thinks that God is going to punish her for being a bad person. She wouldn't say that, but that's what it is. She had a bad childhood. She has extreme anxiety about me and my brother. . . . I have extreme anxiety about my brother and the people I care about and myself. . . . I think it's a learned response from my mother, though I know that the sexual abuse was a major trigger of my fear.
>
> —*Lydia, 23 on how she thinks her mom's mental health struggles affected her*

There is also interesting evidence to suggest that experiences in families going back more than one generation may affect well-being. A series of studies investigating the role of genes, environment, and *transgenerational patterns of stress* help to explain how and why stress "runs in families"—even over several generations. Scholars such as Michael Meaney and Moshe Szyf have dedicated more than 40 years of research to understanding this exchange, a phenomenon called "epigenetics."

Epigenetics refers to the study of how various factors, such as age, disease, environment, or lifestyle influence how genes are "expressed"—or turned on or off, if you will. For instance, traumatic experience in one's personal *or familial* past leave a molecular signature at the DNA level.[4] What does this mean? People who grew up in stressful, traumatic, or abusive environments carry more than just memories. These experiences become part of their genetic makeup, which is then passed down to their children and even their children's children.[5] Timing matters too—being exposed to trauma as a child leads to more DNA changes than being exposed to trauma as an adult. This means that all of us inherit more than just the physical, intellectual, or sensory characteristics of our ancestors; we inherit the emotional and cognitive impact of their experiences—positive and negative.[6]

Family lineages pass on more than stress, though—they pass on *strengths* as well. These strengths, along with whatever extra supports are available in our environments (e.g., nurturing caretakers, effective therapy, positive friends, supportive school environments, etc.), can also alter our DNA.[7] All of this suggests that the high emotional reactivity; tendency toward negative, fear-based thinking; and skewed perceptions (seeing high threat where there may be little) that you may observe in your child may reflect stress accumulated across generations. Likewise, the particular inner resilience you notice may also reflect intergenerational heartiness. Regardless of what your child may have inherited in this way, though, this research also suggests that whatever we do now to learn resilience-linked skills will add to the family legacy for future generations. This is quite heartening and motivating!

The upshot of current science related to stress is that no matter where it comes from, few of us can escape stress. Learning to healthfully work with emotion, thoughts, and actions can make a difference for individuals and for their future children and even grandchildren.

And the tools needed to understand and enact deep-rooted change have never been more available than they are now. Clinical research has contributed to the development of an increasingly advanced and impressive array of therapeutic tools that help with transforming stress and negativity into wisdom, clarity, and calmness. We'll cover more of these tools and techniques in later chapters.

Impact of Self-Injury on Siblings

The impact of self-injury on siblings can be very powerful. It can also go unnoticed, particularly if siblings are quiet and rarely "rock the boat." How siblings are impacted is quite variable. For example, a few years ago, the brother of a self-injurious young woman (a student at one of our universities) contacted us. His sister had struggled with self-injury and a variety of other challenges for most of their shared adolescence and early adulthood. He had entered college wanting to be a lawyer, but his sister's struggles had inspired him to use his legal interests and skills to specialize in advocacy law for people struggling with mental health challenges. He wanted to come work with us over the summer to better understand self-injury and to launch his policy work in this area. While this young man's fervor was rare, his inspiration is hardly unique. We have talked to dozens of parents, family members, and friends, as well as people who self-injure themselves, who are motivated to help others after witnessing a loved one's struggle with self-injury or dealing with their own.

Unfortunately, the desire to help others is not the most common type of impact that self-injury has on siblings. Siblings are, more often than not, negatively affected by sharing parents and space with a self-injurious sister or brother. Parental attention is often directed to the child who is physically harming his or her body. The heightened stress this poses for parents means less attentive and relaxed time with other children. Moreover, walking into bathrooms or other shared spaces to find blood can be unexpected and disconcerting. Having someone around who is moody and unpredictable, or who periodically causes significant upsets in the

> Siblings are, more often than not, negatively affected by sharing parents and space with a self-injurious sister or brother.

family, such as Emergency Room visits or full meltdowns during family time, can create challenges for sibling health and well-being.

The particular nature of the impact on siblings will depend on factors such as sibling age, relationship quality between family members (including between siblings), duration and intensity of the self-injury, sibling perceptions of parent availability, and parental responses to the self-injury. Providing information about the situation, assuring siblings that parents are still present and connected to *all* their children, taking proactive and useful steps to support the self-injuring child, and expressing both a rational and positive perspective about the future will all be helpful in keeping siblings connected and supported.

In sum, having a sibling who is struggling can pose challenges, but it also provides some opportunities. Greater honesty and authenticity within the family and the process of moving through hardship and into greater stability together, even though harrowing at times, can also bring increased closeness. The more that parents recognize opportunities to educate, authentically connect, and value the connection that comes from co-experiencing hard times, particularly if everyone has adequate support, the more likely it will be that self-injury will not leave lasting family wounds.

Parenting Imbalances

It is important to note that families in which self-injury occurs are very diverse. Parents of individuals who self-injure come in all forms, shapes, colors, and sizes, and reflect the rapidly shifting demographic trends in society overall. Regardless of whether the young person is being actively parented by a single parent or in a blended family spread across one or two or more households, it is not uncommon to see significant differences in how two parents are involved, even if they live in the same house. Most often in two-parent families with a mother and father, the mother describes herself as serving as the "sensitive issues communicator" and the "emotional support." In this case, the mother often knows details about the when, how, where, what, and why of the self-injury as well as what is happening in the daily life of her child that affects his or her emotional and physical state. Fathers are often described by mothers and youth as being less comfortable with initiating emotionally sensitive or vulnerable conversations, or knowing details about their child's emotional state. As one father noted:

> Unfortunately, I did not know she was self-injuring until literally the night we had to meet her at the emergency room. I did not understand; I didn't even have knowledge that this stuff went on. So it was very scary when that happened. It was the doctors that explained it to me. . . . In retrospect, though, I think I might have turned a blind eye; I think I was really in denial or something.
>
> —*Paul, father of a self-injurious adolescent*

It is important to know that while this gender split is the most common in traditional heterosexual parent families (there is no research to indicate whether there are similar patterns in non-heterosexual families), it is not the only pattern. For example, a father in one of our studies described being the first and, until our interview, the only person to know about his son's self-injury. He had decided not to tell his wife out of fear that it might be too much for her to handle. In other families, both parents shared equal knowledge and were as likely as the other to initiate or end up in emotionally arduous conversations with their children.

Some youth—nearly 20%—use self-injury as means of communicating desire for someone to notice them—often this means a yearning for a deeper connection with one or more parents. One study found that youth were more likely to engage in frequent self-injury when their relationships with their fathers were characterized by poor communication and rare acts of love coupled with a high degree of admiration and emulation.[8] Interestingly, another study noted significant increases in the quality of father–child relationships *as a result of* teen self-injury, suggesting that it may, in fact, effectively work to enhance connection—at least in some cases.[9]

> Studies consistently show that self-injurious youth benefit from having both parents (in two-parent families) know about their self-injury and, to the extent possible, provide support.

In applying this to your own family, it is important to be conscious and thoughtful about the roles that each parent plays. Studies consistently show that self-injurious youth benefit from having both parents (in two-parent families) know about their self-injury and, to the extent possible, provide support. And, despite what your teen may say to you, she or he will need your support. Since there is some evidence that self-injury serves as a way for teens to express hard-to-communicate feelings with parents and other important loved ones, it will be helpful to encourage the involvement of family members who might be more remote, such as less or uninvolved parents.

Effects of Parenting a Self-Injurious Child on Your Well-Being: Put Your Own Oxygen Mask on First

In addition to the scars left on the bodies of those who self-injure regularly, parents and other family members are often quiet bearers of the wounds self-injury inflicts. Of parents we have interviewed, 78% indicated that they and their families have experienced emotional hardship (sadness, guilt, grief) as a result of their child's self-injury. Despite the startlingly high prevalence of NSSI in teens and young adults, most families feel alone in dealing with the emotional wounds caused by self-injury. Fear of confiding in others or concerns over possible fallout from confiding in others can leave parents feeling alone. As one of our parents stated:

> It was never an easy subject to talk about. A couple of friends I shared with have never mentioned it again. One friend with a daughter the same age seems to avoid the conversation, almost as if self-injury might somehow be contagious.
>
> —*Carla, on talking about self-injury with other people*

In addition to feeling isolated, parents are often likely to feel stressed. Most of us know that when one member of our family is stressed, the likelihood that the rest of us will feel it and react to it with our own stress is also high. Moreover, parents' own styles of dealing with emotions can interact strongly with their children's styles and inadvertently intensify the underlying risk factors for self-injury. Parents of adolescents with self-injury tend to react to their adolescents' distress by decreasing support and increasing levels of control. It is *very difficult* to stay balanced and warm in the presence of someone who is distressed, seemingly unreasonable, or who seems to be making poor decisions. Supportive, warm, and kind but directive parenting does not always come naturally. Some of the emotional and thought patterns that render youth vulnerable to self-injury may also be experienced by their parents. Thus, the challenges of parenting self-injurious youth can sorely tax parents' capacities.

Secondary Stress

You may have already noticed that we often discuss the role of "secondary stress" on family functioning. This refers to stress caused by being around other people's stress and often by caring for others who are chronically compromised in some way. For example, long-time caregivers of elderly relatives or children with disabilities frequently experience fatigue, worry, and other adverse health conditions as a result of the caregiving they provide. Although we rarely think about it in the same way, research shows that caregivers of youth who are experiencing emotional or psychological challenges experience difficulties similar to those of caregivers of physically or developmentally disabled children or elders. Unlike caregivers for these groups, however, parents of self-injurious teens may experience unique challenges due to the facts that NSSI (1) is not socially visible, but is often chronic; (2) occurs within the context of otherwise *normal development*; and (3) is often episodic, with long periods of silence between episodes.[10]

The episodic nature of NSSI can also heighten feelings of emotional and existential uncertainty. The fact that NSSI can be actively used for days, weeks, or months to deal with stress, but then can be followed by periods of inactivity in which it may seem to be "over" could help explain why parents of children who self-injure often report feeling like they are "walking on eggshells" when interacting with their children. Parents

> Research shows that caregivers of youth who are experiencing emotional or psychological challenges experience difficulties similar to those of caregivers of physically or developmentally disabled children or elders.

have reported that they believe that saying or doing the "wrong thing" will upset their children and lead to another period of self-injury.

For these reasons, a portion of this book focuses on helping parents use a set of tools for managing thoughts and emotions; these are similar to the tools your self-injurious child will be taught. Learning more about how to use present moment awareness, to direct attention to experiences that soothe emotions, and to work with negative thinking patterns will all help you to manage stress, to connect more fully with your child, and to model for your child more positive ways of dealing with stress.

What Can I Expect?

What many parents at the beginning of this phase of their lives do not know is that navigating self-injury actually opens up opportunities for greater closeness, even if not in the short term. A full 66% of parents in one of our studies reported that the experience of having a child who self-injures has brought or will bring them closer together, following up with insights such as these:

> Although not a sharer by nature, this has become the catalyst for communication and conversation and agreement to meet with a therapist weekly.
> —*Shane, on the impact self-injury has had on family communication*

> I think that I have been able to step back from wanting to solve everything for my daughter. I realize that she needs opportunities for success, and that means sometimes having those tough times. I am trying to be a really attentive listener and hear what she is saying rather than thinking that I know what she is saying. I ask more questions and try to put any answers out of my mind. I try to make sure that my girl knows that it is OK to feel whatever she is feeling. My daughter is a sensitive soul and reaches out to me when she senses that I am having some of my own struggles. We were close, but we definitely have become even closer.
> —*Tonya, on the impact self-injury has had on her relationship with her daughter*

Recovery didn't happen overnight so it doesn't change overnight; it takes a lot of work, and it doesn't just take just that individual, it takes the parents understanding, it takes the siblings understanding.

—Lara, on the role of the whole family in self-injury recovery

Knowing that there is likely to be light at the end of the tunnel, however, goes only some of the way in helping parents stay as present, calm, and compassionate as they can for themselves, their children, and other family members. Indeed, parents have the strong tendency to be so focused on securing their children's well-being and support that they don't seek adequate support for themselves. Virtually all parents in our study described feeling sad or unhappy, worried about their children's future, emotionally strained and tired, and that their children's self-injury had taken a significant toll on their families. It's surprising then to hear that so few parents had told others about their challenges. As several parents shared:

My child takes up my time almost 24/7. She has been very hard to treat, as she is allergic and/or resistant to most meds. She depends on me too much I think at times. Until we can find the solution that works for her, I feel I have to put her first.

—Lara, mother to 15-year-old who self-injures

Self-injury is really difficult for most people to relate to. I don't think many people know how to respond. We have no support programs for the self-injurer or the parents in my location. It is a quiet epidemic.

—Shane, on self-injury stigma

Every parent with whom we have spoken about a child's self-injury clearly communicates care and concern. Not all parents, however, possess the same resources for helping their children. Differences in availability of skilled treatment, cost of treatment and/or differences in insurance coverage, and differing levels of other stresses and inner resources all contribute to parent capacity to help a struggling child. Stigma associated with seeking treatment can also be a big barrier since some families view seeing a therapist as a sign of personal or family failure.

Moreover, the road to full recovery can be long. The effectiveness of professional treatment and other supports is strongly affected by *child readiness to change,* how much they've come to rely on self-injury for coping, and availability of other key resources (such as therapy) needed to stop the behavior. All of these factors matter and change over time in ways that can help or frustrate everyone involved. Nevertheless, if you are reading this, then rest assured that you have the most important tools needed for the road ahead: your love, concern, and a willingness to stay engaged.

Activities

Family Strengths Activity

We often forget to focus on the strengths we have at our disposal to overcome challenges. This questionnaire is designed to help you think honestly and accurately about your family's strengths. Don't worry about the areas in which you score lower than you might like. This book is designed to provide you with tools and resources for developing and supporting the areas assessed here.

This exercise has two parts: First, you and your child who is engaging in self-injury will each separately complete a copy of the questionnaire that follows. Second, we would like you to spend a few minutes talking with one another about your answers and where your ratings are similar and different. We've provided suggestions for this conversation and debriefing.

Part 1: Parent and Youth Assessment

Parent Questionnaire

Directions: Please read each statement and decide how often/to what degree each statement is true of your family (1 = Never, 2 = Rarely, 3 = Somewhat, 4 = Often, 5 = Almost Always).

_____1. We enjoy talking to one another.

_____2. Our family recognizes when a problem exists.

_____3. Our family handles stress well.

_____4. Our family can come up with solutions to easily resolve problems.

_____5. We feel comfortable sharing our affection with one another.

_____6. Everyone gets a say in family decisions.

_____7. It is easy for us to work together to overcome crises in our family.

_____8. We can effectively talk to each other even when we are upset.

_____9. We give praise when someone has done something positive.

_____10. When we ask someone in our family to do something, they do it.

_____11. We have enjoyable memories with one another.

_____12. We often confide in each other.

_____13. We are committed to supporting our family's well-being.

_____14. Family members do not have trouble meeting their responsibilities.

_____15. We feel a strong connection with one another.

_____16. We discuss things before decisions that affect the whole family are made.

_____17. We are respectful to each other when someone is expressing a different point of view.

_____18. We are sensitive to other family member's feelings.

_____19. We trust each other.

_____20. We support one another even when someone has made a bad decision.

_____21. We are kind to one another.

_____22. We do not put each other down.

_____23. We support family members, even when we disagree with them.

_____24. Our family has fun together.

Child Questionnaire

Directions: Please read each statement and decide how often/ to what degree each is true of your family (1 = Never, 2 = Rarely, 3 = Somewhat, 4 = Often, 5 = Almost Always).

_____ 1. We enjoy talking to one another.

_____ 2. Our family recognizes when a problem exists.

_____ 3. Our family handles stress well.

_____ 4. Our family can come up with solutions to easily resolve problems.

_____ 5. We feel comfortable sharing our affection with one another.

_____ 6. Everyone gets a say in family decisions.

_____ 7. It is easy for us to work together to overcome crises in our family.

_____ 8. We can effectively talk to each other even when we are upset.

_____ 9. We give praise when someone has done something positive.

_____ 10. When we ask someone in our family to do something, they do it.

_____ 11. We have enjoyable memories with one another.

_____ 12. We often confide in each other.

_____ 13. We are committed to supporting our family's well-being.

_____ 14. Family members do not have trouble meeting their responsibilities.

_____ 15. We feel a strong connection with one another.

_____ 16. We discuss things before decisions that affect the whole family are made.

_____ 17. We are respectful to each other when someone is expressing a different point of view.

_____ 18. We are sensitive to other family member's feelings.

_____ 19. We trust each other.

_____ 20. We support one another even when someone has made a bad decision.

_____ 21. We are kind to one another.

_____ 22. We do not put each other down.

_____ 23. We support family members, even when we disagree with them.

_____ 24. Our family has fun together.

Part 2: Conversation and Debriefing

Discuss where you are similar or different and why you think this may be the case. Pick out 1–2 areas where you agree on a strength. Pick out 1–2 areas where you agree that you would like to work on some changes. Feel free to give this questionnaire to other family members as well!

No family is perfect, but this questionnaire can help you identify the strengths of your family (also called "resilience") as well as challenge areas. It can be helpful to think about these strengths during times of crisis, so that you can come up with the best strategies for coping.

Research shows that strong, stable families have certain qualities. These include:

- Open, effective communication
- Expressions of affection and warmth
- Comfort in talking with each other
- Respect
- Sense of connectedness and belonging
- Problem-solving skills
- Support and encouragement
- Cooperation and loyalty
- Commitment to helping each other

When families are dealing with self-injury, it is especially important to balance the understanding of risk factors with what families are doing "right." For example, one family scores high on the expressions of affection and warmth, but also scores low on problem-solving. Another family may score high on commitment to helping each other, but may lack open and effective communication. Understanding family strengths provides useful information that can help families improve relationships. Research has shown that teens are less likely to self-injure when their families have *open communication, are comfortable talking* to one another, are *respectful* of one another, and express affection. Good communication allows family members to share their own perspectives and to feel "heard," which leads to a *sense of connectedness and belonging.*

Youth who self-injure often feel isolated. *Support and encouragement* from family members (praise, compliments) can increase the sense of loyalty and commitment, which can help to foster resilience in self-injurious youth.

The Family Strengths Activity is designed to help you identify family strengths (those characteristics of your family that you rated as "often" or "almost always"). Take pride in these! If your results are very different from those of your teen *OR* if you both feel that your family is low on strengths, consider seeking professional assistance from a trained family therapist.

Reflection Activity: Common Problems in Families of Teens Who Self-Injure

Here you will find a list of common problems that families of teens who self-injure may encounter. We encourage you to review this list and check those that you believe apply to your situation. As you proceed through this book, you will find that we discuss each of these areas and provide information, strategies, and suggestions for moving forward.

Teenager Function and Behavior
My teen doesn't seem to have any friends.
My teen doesn't leave his or her room anymore.
Some of my teen's friends appear to be bad influences.

Parent Distress
I worry more than ever now.
I have difficulty talking to my friends about what's really going on in my life.
My friends ignore what is happening with my teen.
My friends aren't aware of what is happening.
I worry about upsetting my teen.
I worry that my child will never get better.
I feel that I've let my child down because I'm not able to protect him or her from this.
I feel helpless.
My life feels like it is falling apart.
I can't take much more of this.

Family and Marital Issues
Our family doesn't get along well any more.
We don't talk about what's going on.
I have no time for my other children and my spouse.
Our household feels so tense all of the time.
My spouse/partner and I do not share the burden of this equally.
I feel that my marriage is strained.
My teen's condition is becoming a financial burden.

Healthcare or School System Issues
I don't know how to get the information I want.
I have difficulties communicating with school staff.
I have difficulties communicating with my teen's therapist.

The Context of Self-Injury

Where Did It Come From?

At the moment, transforming and enhancing our bodies is a major American cultural imperative supported by both commerce and medicine. "Body modification" businesses operate in most cities and towns; teenage girls are sporting belly-button jewelry and eyebrow rings. The growing popularity of such "body projects"—ranging from garden-variety piercing and tattooing to bizarre forms of cosmetic surgery—suggests a new mind-set about the malleability of the body as well as its ability to withstand violation and penetration. For many in the younger generation, not just those who think of themselves as "Goth," the body is a critical message board, a way to convey information about the self.

—Joan Jacobs Brumberg (1998)

Setting the Stage: Self-Injury in Context

Self-injury did not arise in a vacuum. In fact, it is only one of many signs that youth and adults living in contemporary times are struggling. Rates of mental health disorders among adults in the United States are some of the highest in the world, with one in four adults living with a mental health disorder.[1] Rates for youth are similar, with 22% of teens experiencing mental health symptoms severe enough to interfere with daily functioning.[2] A large majority of these mental health issues are related to difficulties managing or otherwise regulating emotions, such as anxiety, mood, and behavior disorders. In addition, there are the many other challenges that teens face, such as disordered eating, substance use, and issues related to sexuality. In short, healthy, happy, well-adjusted, and functioning teens are more difficult than ever to locate.

We also have to consider the contexts within which people live. As researcher and historian Joan Brumberg and self-injury treatment specialist Wendy Lader have each pointed out, the rise and acceptance of body modification over the past several decades may well have paved the way for a full-scale emergence of self-injury as a form of emotional self-expression.[3] The late 1980s ushered in a broad fascination with *the body as a canvas for self-expression* that fundamentally changed the way youth used their bodies, not just clothing or makeup, to express everything from group affiliation to anxiety. Joan Brumberg, who authored the book, *The Body Project*, described the widespread rise of tattooing and piercing as further reifying the body as a canvas that could be sculpted through more than simple manipulation of fat and muscle. It could literally and figuratively be used to express identity, art, social affiliation, or states of mind, such as anxiety, desire, and depression. Ink, piercings, blades, burners, even fingernails transformed body tissue from a simple part of oneself to a billboard or beacon that could be used to communicate with the world.

> The late 1980s ushered in a broad fascination with *the body as a canvas for self-expression* that fundamentally changed the way youth used their bodies, not just clothing or makeup, to express everything from group affiliation to anxiety.

In addition to the heightened focus on body and self, the end of the past century and new millennium has been described as the entryway to the age of "extreme" everything—sports, drinks, food portions, alcohol consumption—hedonism in all forms. The motto, "if a little is good, more is better" is an apt reflection of the modern age. Interestingly, the current era is also a time of high disclosure. Mainstream culture and media outlets expanded from offering current events and fictional stories to "reality" television shows. Perhaps not surprisingly, it was during the 1990s that more than a dozen pop icons disclosed having used self-injury as a way to cope with stress. Celebrities such as Johnny Depp, Angelina Jolie, Princess Diana, Christina Ricci, and a number of others appeared in mainstream media over the course of this decade to share experiences in which self-injury featured prominently. They were not advocating it in most cases, but they were talking about their troubles in ways that were raw, human, and very easy to identify with. Perhaps because of this, the behavior began making its way into popular culture through movies, songs, books, music, and news media. The United States went from no news stories mentioning self-injury in the early 1980s to more than 300 unique reports of the phenomenon by 2006.[4] By the first decade of the new millennium, self-injury made regular appearances in sympathetic characters and lives featured in movies, TV shows, music, and poetry. And, once the Internet made its debut, self-injury joined dozens of other behaviors and activities that could be discussed online and in text, video, and interactive forums. In short, it's not hard to understand how self-injury may have entered the popular imagination as a practice for reducing or expressing stress or disconnecting from the present situation.

Is Self-Injury Spreading?

For the past 10 years or so, self-injury has been called "the next teen disorder." Like eating disorders, which gained a lot of attention in the late 1980s and early 1990s, self-injury without suicidal intent seemed to emerge from relative obscurity into the mainstream almost overnight. Prior to 2000, the behavior was documented largely in youth and adults, mainly women, with clear mental health challenges. If self-injury was discussed among health professionals at all, it was usually related to self-destructive personality issues and/or a history of trauma—sexual abuse in particular. However, the past decade saw a flood of reports from professionals who work with children in schools, adolescent health clinics, and youth programs that suggest that self-injury had begun to "spread"—inside and outside of the United States.

We will never know for sure whether the prevalence of self-injury has actually increased or whether *awareness* of the behavior increased (or some combination of both). While we have little information available on the incidence of self-injury prior to the early part of the millennium, there is good reason to believe that widespread self-injury may be relatively unique to current generations of youth.

What Does Being a Teen Have to Do with It?

> *I was very melodramatic and depressed all the time. I got the idea of cutting by the Internet, probably. Reading or chat rooms I guess, but I don't even remember if it was a natural idea or not. That's probably the last time I had suicidal thoughts, but I did not self-injure to die. It was more like surface cuts. I would also restrict my diet and not eat and things like that because I was really concerned about weight. I went on birth control and got depressed, and so I stopped the birth control and started cutting myself again. Then I broke up with my boyfriend at the time and that did not help at all.*
>
> —Sophie, on her self-injury

In many ways, the stage of life we identify as adolescence is itself a risk factor for self-injury. This period of life is also the most common for the onset of most major mental disorders. Much of this stems from the rapid and complex brain and physical development occurring at this time. Indeed, adolescence is second only to the first 2 years of life in the changes taking place in both the body and brain, including the development and refinement of synapses in the brain. Unlike early childhood, however, in which the extent of physical growth is obvious, much of the development occurring in the adolescent years— be it psychological, social, moral, cognitive, sexual, and spiritual—is largely invisible.

The many physical, neurological, and identity-linked changes taking place leave adolescents *very* sensitive to emotional experiences.[5]

They are most influenced by interactions with others. Experiences such as social rejection and acceptance have the capability to strongly influence the adolescent sense of self-value and esteem. Adolescents tend to feel all emotions, especially negative emotions, more acutely than they do as children or as adults. As some might describe, they are "sensitive." Some of these feelings are experienced as overwhelming and have profound and often exaggerated inner effects. Behaviors that may be effective in the short term but maladaptive in the long run, such as self-injury or substance abuse, are common during this time. If trauma, biological imbalances, or challenging environments are also included, there are likely to be additional harmful consequences or delays to healthy development.

> Adolescents tend to feel all emotions, especially negative emotions, more acutely than they do as children or as adults.

Self-injury may have developmentally symbolic value as well. Some adolescents report that they use self-injury as a way to express their fear or discomfort with conflicts within themselves. These conflicts often relate to autonomy and connection, physical changes in their bodies and sexual impulses, individual mastery, social belonging, and other key areas of development. Self-injury may also act as a physical and metaphorical attempt to integrate spirit, body, and psyche. Some people even describe self-injury as a transcendent act: one capable of granting authenticity and a sense of physical, mental, emotional, and spiritual equilibrium—even if this is felt only fleetingly.[6] *The particular attractiveness of self-injury to adolescents may lie in its capacity to serve as a vehicle for expression of pain as well as a striving toward wholeness.* We emphasize this here because the impulse from which self-injury often comes is fundamentally understandable and life-oriented. The desire to feel better is healthy and can be used as the basis for building more positive outlets to accomplishing this end.

Self-Injury and Social Media

My self-injury definitely worsened after the Internet came along. There were so many chat rooms for people who self-injured. It did help in the short term but not in the long term. I have to avoid on-

line self-injury communities now because they are so triggering.

—Heather, 20, on the contribution of social media to her
self-injury

The technological changes taking place at the end of the past century seemed to go into hyperdrive with the dawn of the new millennium. Now, almost two decades past the turn of the century, it is clear to us that we have, indeed, entered the age of constant connection. For those of us born well before the turn of the past century, it can be difficult to identify with youth coming of age today. Their time is so different from many of the experiences that shaped their parents' upbringings: wall-connected telephones, busy signals, TVs with five channels and no remote, turntables, cars with manually operated windows, a lot of unstructured time, boredom, even simply going outside to play.

In 1975, most American families owned or had access to a television, a radio, a phone, and a mailbox. Some received newspapers. By 2006, media routes into and out of the average American home had nearly tripled. Not only had technologies for these basic 1975 media modalities expanded considerably with the advent of cable, satellite, VHS and DVD, and "express" mail deliveries, development of wholly novel technologies evolved as well. By 2017, the routes into and out of the average home have become so diffuse that researchers stopped counting and simply identified them as the "Internet of things." As the Pew Foundation has consistently reported in its tracking of our online lives,[7] the vast majority of youth and adults live in homes that are connected to the Internet—usually through multiple devices (computers, smartphones, tablets, game consoles, readers, and so on). This means that most young people (and adults) possess unparalleled opportunities to connect while at the same time feeling very disconnected from one another.

> Most young people (and adults) possess unparalleled opportunities to connect while at the same time feeling very disconnected from one another.

In many ways, youth live in what we have come to think of as the *connectedness paradox*—the experience of being simultaneously overconnected to others while also underconnected to developmentally supportive resources. For example, it is possible to have hundreds of Facebook friends and even more Snapchat or Instagram followers but to have very few individuals with whom one can share private thoughts or feelings. Indeed, analysis of the 2014 UCLA college freshman survey,[8] an annual survey now in its 50th year of administration, showed that the amount of time students report socializing with friends during their final year of high school has continued to steadily decline. In 1987, 37.9% of incoming college students socialized at least 16 hours per week with friends. In 2014, this declined to only 18% of students. In contrast and not surprisingly, students report spending more time interacting with others through online social networks. Since 2007, the percentage of students dedicating 6 hours or more per week to social media increased from 18.9% to 27.2%. While we cannot necessarily link this shift to young people's well-being directly, it is important to note that the same 2014 analysis of the UCLA freshman survey documented the lowest emotional health ratings (50.7% reported good emotional health) since the survey started. Additionally, the proportion of students who "frequently" felt depressed rose to 9.5%, 3.4 percentage points higher than in 2009, when this figure reached its lowest point.

One of the core components of the connectedness paradox is the fact that we have entered a time of unparalleled focus on the "self" as a projected identity that sometimes bears little resemblance to one's real life. In other words, teens and young adults now struggle with how different their "true selves" are from how they portray themselves online. This part of the new age is truly fascinating. During no time in history have human beings seen pictures of their own faces and (especially) bodies as they do now. Think about it—you may have looked in a mirror a few times a day at most and probably stopped noticing the pictures that your parents may have had up in the house once the novelty wore off. Today's average teen spends large amounts of time not only *looking* at his or her own image but also *generating a countless number of new, critically assessed self-images* to post and view almost daily. Social media venues actively encourage continued generation and scrutiny of "self" in ways that constantly refocus attention on what one looks like. Unfortunately, this societal focus on oneself impacts adolescents particularly hard, given that they often already struggle with physical appearance, how they fit in, and the stress resulting from this.

Perhaps the most potent element of the digital age, and one every parent needs to be aware of, has been the advent of social media. Social media are defined as websites and applications that allow users to create and share content or to participate in social networking. Finding an adolescent today who does not participate in social media would be a true feat. A few common examples of high use among teens include Instagram, Snapchat, Facebook, Twitter, Tumblr, Googl #, and Yik Yak (there are many more, these are just a few very common examples as of the writing of this book). There are also dedicated Internet and app-based communities where users exchange information and bond around particular topic areas. Beyond the tremendous diversity of function (sending images, text, sound) and versatility (e.g., messages that disappear a few seconds after they are sent), a wide variety of content is posted and exchanged on these sites. Although these can be sources of self-expression and social support, they are also places where:

- *Emotional stakes can be high.* How others respond to posts matters a lot to many youth (and adult!) users. An unfavorable or low positive response from online connections can affect mood and feelings of well-being in offline life. The number of "likes" someone receives, neutral or negative feedback, or even lack of response to posts/shares can seriously ruin a teen's day. For depressed or anxious youth, this can trigger a downward spiral.
- *Users can become targets of bullying.* Cyberbullying has come to be something all parents know and fear. Bullying can be overt (outright threats or derogatory statements) or more subtle (small jabs or put downs). Part of what makes it so much more potent than the experiences most contemporary parents had as kids is the social element of it all. Most hurtful comments can be seen by a large digital audience and can be delivered with impunity since the digital nature of it all allows for people to demonstrate mean-spiritedness without any human contact at all and without having to witness the emotional response of the victim.
- *Content shared can be triggering.* Much of what is shared by teens online or digitally can be very triggering. Triggers

can include posts of self-injury imagery, accounts of abuse or other victim stories that inspire painful feelings or memories, reminders of loss (such as remaining connected via social media to ex-partners), and feelings of jealousy due to negative self-comparison. People's lives tend to look perfect in social media portrayals, so it is easy for youth to assume they are the lone failures. Experiences like these can all trigger the feelings that lead to self-injury or other self-harming behaviors.

- *Communities are organized around self-injury, and these can help or hurt recovery.* It is important for you to know that there are many digital gathering spaces specific to self-injury (and eating disorders and any other behavior, practice, or perspective you can think of). While many of the self-injury–specific communities can be found in social media, they can also be found as commenters on YouTube self-injury videos or gathered in self-injury message boards. Studies show that some of these gatherings can be helpful and supportive, but some can overtly or inadvertently trigger self-injury behavior.

- *Constant access may enable triggering or reinforcing peer exchanges.* The dependence of youth (and many adults) on connecting with peers on social media, combined with difficulty in controlling impulses, means that teens may not be able to stop themselves from being in frequent connection with triggering content. Sleep deprivation and lack of true "down time" can make the effects of this exposure much worse. In addition, teens who self-injure are more likely to have friends who also injure and struggle with other mental health challenges. So, this puts them at additional risk of having peer relationships that lead to more self-injury episodes and thus reinforces a cycle of behavior.

In short, it is clear that changes in technology have allowed unprecedented access to people, knowledge, and support. It has also posed some challenges. Studies of the effects of sharing self-injury content with others reveal a complex picture. On the one hand, it is clear that individuals who injure can and often do use social media to feel less alone and to solicit support and constructive advice. On the other hand, virtual communities and sharing may introduce, reinforce, and support the very behavior they target.

Why Did This Happen?

The search for the *particular* set of life circumstances and personality characteristics that lead a *particular* person to self-injure has not been terribly fruitful. It is important to note that understanding the origins of common forms of NSSI in adolescence is complicated. The question of *why* boils down to this: someone who struggles to cope with negative emotions has found self-injury to be helpful in this regard. But that does not tell us much of use, does it? The stories of different people's experiences of negative emotions is wide ranging and varied.

> The question of *why* boils down to this: someone who struggles to cope with negative emotions has found self-injury to be helpful in this regard.

The complexity and rapid nature of developmental changes taking place during adolescence create an environment full of both risk factors and protective factors. For example, friends who seem like negative influences at the outset may end up providing much needed social support later on. Prolonged periods of moodiness and depression may offer opportunity for reflection and give way to major self-realizations (for instance, think of a young person struggling to accept that he or she is gay/lesbian/transgender). Remember that there are two sides to every coin; this allows us to open our minds to the possibility of hope where there may have been only darkness.

Despite the fact that it is so difficult to answer fully, *why* is the most common question that parents have and one we will address in detail next. Many of the factors we discuss in Chapter 4 can be viewed as both risk and protective factors.

Activities

Parent–Teen Reflection and Communication Activity

Please take some time to sit down and talk with your teen using the following questions as prompts. They are designed to inspire conversation about the material from this chapter in a deep and personal way.

1. What is different about your teen's environment compared to when you were growing up? How does this influence your parenting?

2. How does the use of social media help and hurt growing up in today's culture?

3. How has the Internet affected your teen's thinking about self-injury? How does he or she feel when coming across content that may trigger urges to self-injure?

4. How do you think time should be structured around surfing the Internet? What are the pros and cons of setting up more rules around the use of social media?

Where It Starts and Why It Works

I have come a long way in accepting that there are no answers to the big "whys" of adversities and suffering. If we can accept this, we can feel so much more peace with what is, despite what we don't know.

—Harriet Cabelly, author of *Living Well Despite Adversity*[1]

Well, it certainly worked in the short term. Yeah. I wish that it could have only been that superficial cutting. You can't help but be reminded of it. You want to move on. You want to feel like an adult, a mature person who can handle themselves, and you don't want to have physical evidence of the fact that you can't. . . . I wonder what I would have done if I didn't do that. I honestly don't know that I have an answer for that—I don't know what I would have done. I wish my environment had not been what it was. I wish I'd had somebody to talk to.

—Mary, reflections on her self-injury at age 24

Isn't Self-Injury Unnatural?

Many people have a hard time understanding how others could choose to inflict pain on themselves. Most people think of pain as something to avoid, to move away from. But we all have had experiences of pain feeling good in some way as well. Perhaps it's that itch that needs to be scratched during a bout of poison ivy or the soreness you feel when you've pushed your muscles to their limit running that last hill. Pain in these cases can lead to feelings of satisfaction, relief, or accomplishment. Although self-injury is not quite the same as these examples, it does come from the same desire to push through the hurt in order to feel better. Thus, contrary to what it may look like or what many believe, nonsuicidal self-injury (NSSI) is generally life *preserving* in intent.

In this way, self-injury is paradoxical in nature. What brings physical pain is actually an outlet for immediate expression and relief of emotional pain. In J. K. Rowling's book, *The Casual Vacancy*, a teenage girl's cutting episode is explained this way: "The blade drew the pain away from her screaming thoughts and transmuted it into animal burning of nerves and skin; relief and release in every cut." This description highlights the two most common reasons science tells us that adolescents self-injure: (1) to express and control painful or overwhelming emotions and (2) to escape or avoid feelings of emptiness or numbness.

Understanding *why* your teen self-injures will allow you to move beyond feeling hopeless to focusing on what you can do to support your child and your family. Let's turn now to reviewing what current science tells us about how self-injury works to soothe.

Why Self-Injure?

This question encompasses three distinct parts:

1. What life factors help to explain why young people initiate self-injury in the first place?
2. What kinds of events tend to precipitate self-injury episodes?
3. Why does self-injury work once it is started?

It is important to reiterate that there is no single path to self-injury. The factors that go into making self-injury a regular part of someone's life are quite variable and come together for individuals in unique ways. Science helps us to understand the general trends and most striking or common patterns but cannot tell us much about why any particular person self-injures.

Understanding what motivates *your* child to engage in self-injury is a complex task but crucial for helping your teen to liberate herself. It may be that some childhood events felt overwhelming (e.g., a death in the family, a hard move, or parental divorce); that your child experienced some sort of chronic hardship, abuse, or trauma; or that she simply feels emotions more deeply and reacts more intensely than others seem to. Reviewed here is our most common understanding about why individuals self-injure. While we cannot explain every path to self-injury, this is a good place to start.

> Understanding what motivates *your* child to engage in self-injury is a complex task but crucial for helping your teen to liberate herself.

Why Start Self-Injuring in the First Place?

Understanding the factors that contribute to initiating self-injury in the first place is challenging. Nevertheless, questions such as "where did this start" and/or "what happened in my child's life to cause this?" are some of the most common we encounter from parents. Sometimes, as we discussed in the previous chapter, there are no obvious explanations. Often, however, there are precipitating events or periods of hardship, in families or in your child's life alone, that set the stage for self-injury and/or other adverse behaviors. What we have identified here are the most common external factors reported by individuals who self-injure. Very few individuals possess *all* of these risk factors, but these are common enough among individuals who self-injure to make them recognize risk factors in the scientific literature.

In some cases, self-injury is strongly linked to a history of sexual abuse and/or poor attachment to parents. It is true that youth with a history of abuse or trauma (such as loss of a parent) or chronic stress (economic hardship due to divorce or other factors) are at significantly higher risk for self-injury than are those who have not experienced these challenges.[2] Why are these so connected? It likely has to do with the fact that emotional and/or sexual abuse (whether it occurs within or outside of the family) during the childhood years often results in the tendency to self-criticize or self-blame. In the face of stressful events, adolescents who have developed this negative way of thinking about themselves may be more likely to engage in NSSI as a way to punish themselves physically. Stories like Linda's, now 23, are relatively common:

> **Linda:** The sexual abuse was so young, but I can't really distinguish a time before it happened. It was multiple incidences, for 2 years, from [ages] 5–7. It was my uncle who lived with my grandmother. He was borderline mentally retarded. And it must have happened a lot the second year because that was the year we stayed with my grandmother because my mother went back to work. Before that it was sporadically at times when the whole family was over—holidays.
>
> **Interviewer:** And your parents found out?
>
> **Linda:** I told them when I was 7. Something was done right away, and they believed me. It has made me a much healthier survivor of it than many other people because it was instant reassurance and affirmation.

Early challenging family experiences can also lead to insecure or poor *attachment to parents*. There is a large body of research on attachment showing that processes or events that interfere with the parent–child bond can be problematic for child *and* parent.[3] Children function best in the world when they are certain of a parent's love, capacity to accommodate and handle the challenges that come along with child-rearing, and when there are regular patterns and expectations in family life. Families in which there is (or was) large or chronic change, parental instability or lack of availability, disruption in routine, and/or unstable or rigid expectations can disrupt children's sense of stability and predictability and their sense of trust. While some children possess the inner resources to navigate these changes and remain strongly connected to parents, not all children do. Furthermore, not all parents are well-equipped to effectively reassure children of their love and presence.

It is important to note that the need for being assured of love, connection to others, routine, and positive and achievable expectations does not end with childhood. Adolescents *and* adults (including parents) do best in the world when they possess the basic qualities of love and connection that come from continual experiences of safety and trust. Parents who have experienced chronic disruption, stress, trauma, or disconnection to key others (e.g., their own parents) at any point in life will be less well-positioned to provide these qualities to their own children and to experience the resulting reciprocal love and care that comes back to them from children. This dynamic, sometimes generations old, can be played out in poignant and painful ways in families of youth who injure.

> Adolescents *and* adults (including parents) do best in the world when they possess the basic qualities of love and connection that come from continual experiences of safety and trust.

We also know that youth who self-injure are more likely than their non–self-injurious peers to come from families where there is parental history of mental health challenges.[4] Linda's mother, for example, struggled with bipolar disorder and was often depressed and even suicidal. Linda felt a deep need to protect and take care of her mother at a very young age. The weight of this perceived responsibility, combined with Linda's fears that she, too, would struggle like her mom did and the events of her childhood (sexual abuse), all left her feeling very overwhelmed by adolescence.

These issues are echoed in science as well. Having a parent experiencing mental health challenges also heightens the risk of a teen experiencing challenges.[5] This can occur through lack of consistent attention and monitoring. For example, a depressed or anxious parent may require more sleep or time alone. It can also occur because of a parent having difficulties being emotionally available and warm, or through social modeling of less than effective ways of dealing with stress, such as alcohol or prescription drug abuse. And, as we discussed in the previous chapter, these children may have inherited a genetic predisposition for mental challenges themselves.

Individuals with another mental health condition, particularly disordered eating, depression, or anxiety, are also at higher than average risk of self-injury. Indeed, having a co-occurring mental health condition is a stronger predictor of self-injury than engaging in other risky behaviors such as recreational drug or alcohol use. On the other hand, the reverse is true also. The presence of self-injury is a risk factor for developing other mental health conditions. This is because many of the mental health conditions that tend to come along with self-injury share underlying difficulties with regulating intense emotions (see this chapter's Science Spotlight).

What Teens Say About Why It Started

When we ask those who injure why they started, they are often unable to identify exactly what triggered it. In reflecting on where it started for her, Siang noted that, in retrospect, self-injury emerged from a mix of early "social modeling" by family members mixed with strong feelings that she did not know how to manage in other ways:

> I think it goes back to my parents, what I went through in childhood. When I was a kid, my brother and I were sent to the states to live with my aunt and uncle to study while my parents stayed in Taiwan. So it's not like abuse or neglect or anything but just the fact of being away from my parents—that really hurt me a lot. But, I didn't really know it back then because I was so young. So as I grew up . . . I think I had a lot of that kind of hidden inside, but I never understood it. In the past few years, I have actually thought about it: where did I learn this violent behavior? I think it was my uncle when I was younger, even before I came to the states. He had these anger outbursts and when we would go visit my grandparents, he would punch stuff. He had a lot of holes in his house, too. I think that's how I learned it. That's how I learned it was okay to have these weird things going on.
>
> —*Siang, age 20, on starting to self-injure*

As reflected in Siang's comment, it can take a while for a young person to sort out all of the early or original experiences, feelings, and/or events that laid the groundwork for self-injury. It is often not until late adolescence, early adulthood, or even beyond that individuals possess the maturity and cognitive ability for this kind of reflection. When we ask young people to identify why they started in the first place, they are most likely to identify more "proximal" (immediate or easy to identify) reasons, such as, "I was just upset and decided to try it," "I was angry at myself or someone else," or, in some cases, "because I wanted someone to notice or be shocked or hurt."

Sadly, we hear stories from a growing number of youth who have no identifiable risk factors in their pasts. Many come from stable and loving families living in strong communities and schools. For these teens, the contemporary commonness of the behavior and the extent to which it is part of the stories, videos, music, or other narratives that today's youth see and hear about growing up seems to be the primary risk factor. This can be very confusing for parents, other adults, and therapists. As one parent shared,

> I felt like our family had so many strengths, I have a pretty happy marriage, three beautiful children who love each other, few traumas in our lives compared to many, and here we are being labeled a "complicated family" with all three children having done some self-harm and two who I fear may not manage. How do I not feel responsible?
>
> —*Shelly, parent of a self-injurious youth*

Similarly, modern culture has also created a group of young people who experiment with self-injury out of curiosity, because they have a friend or sibling or even parent with self-injury experience, and have come to identify with the behavior in some way. In these cases, the doorway into self-injury may have few identifiable risk factors but may, instead, be reflective of peer culture, identity exploration, and experiencing strong emotions.

What Triggers a Self-Injury Episode?

Environmental Triggers

Regardless of how someone arrives at self-injury, the triggers for engaging in a self-injury "episode" (which may be brief or take more time and consist of one or more wounds) are often very consistent. *Triggers* are often events that put an individual at great risk for unhealthy behaviors such as self-injury. Social scientists discuss the causes of behavior in terms of both *distal* (far away) and *proximal* (closer in time) influences. The most commonly identified distal triggers for self-injury include loss or conflict in relationships whether involving family, partner, or peers; abuse by a family member or partner; experience of academic or extracurricular performance difficulties; exposure to others who self-injure; or being under the influence of drugs or alcohol. As experienced therapist Barent Walsh points out, the more complicated an individual's history and family context, the more susceptible he or she may be to reacting to negative experiences through self-injury.[6]

> The more complicated an individual's history and family context, the more susceptible he or she may be to reacting to negative experiences through self-injury.

As you would expect, these upsetting distal events can lead to qualitative changes in who we are and how we view life. These experiences can inspire a sense of failure, self-doubt, frustrated desire, or loss, all of which are considered more proximal self-injury triggers. Perhaps as a result of traumatic earlier experiences, the way that looming deadlines are perceived, pressure to perform (common in athletes), failure to perform as desired or expected, or even endings of any sort (for example, Linda mentioned that movie endings were a trigger for her at times) can all be proximal self-injury triggers.

Urges as Triggers

Triggers for self-injury can also include thoughts or feelings that can lead to urges to self-injure. Urges are a thought, desire, or craving to do something; in this case, to harm oneself. Strong urges can be a common experience for those who self-injure, particularly once someone has injured multiple times. Urges are considered proximal triggers because they are typically close in time to when self-injury occurs. Sometimes, it may feel as though this strong urge to injure comes out of nowhere, a fact that can be upsetting and lead to the desire to injure as a way of diminishing the urge. We'll talk more about accepting and managing urges in later chapters, but for now let's learn more about why, once self-injury starts, it can be so hard to stop.

Tracking the Trigger–Injury Cycle

While this can be tricky for caretakers who often feel like they are walking on eggshells, understanding the way the cycle works is a critical step in learning how to notice and celebrate the moments when typical triggers *do not* lead to self-injury. Learning to pay particular attention to the immediate triggers and consequences of a self-injury episode means asking questions such as: What events cause the desire to injure? When does it usually happen? What self-injury forms are used, and what areas of the body are affected? What happens immediately after, and later? When self-injury is successfully avoided, even when a trigger is present, what happened to make this possible? For someone on the outside looking in, it can be difficult to determine the specific trigger that leads to the injury (or what deters it), particularly since *some* individuals who self-injure will plan for days in advance their self-harm. For this reason, getting to the bottom of triggers for an episode of self-injury can be challenging and may be helped by recording or keeping a diary (both caretakers and individuals who injure can do this; it can be helpful to compare notes; see "Tracking Triggers and the Immediate Consequences Using the ABC's" at the end of this chapter).

Why Does Self-Injury Work? Unpacking the Bio-Psycho-Social Model of Self-Injury

Physical health, mental health, and illness are influenced by many shared factors. The "bio-psycho-social model" is a widely used concept in medicine that asserts that biological, psychological, and social factors are all involved in the causes, course, and outcomes of health and disease. In other words, individuals' genetic makeup and predispositions (biology); their emotions, thoughts, and behaviors (psychology); and their families and social and cultural environments (social) all contribute to health and disease. Importantly, these three domains do not operate independently but instead overlap with and regularly affect one another, as you'll see next. For our purposes, the bio-psycho-social model, first applied to self-injury by Barent Walsh, serves also as a useful tool for organizing and understanding the various factors that contribute to the development and continuation of self-injury.[7] At the end of this chapter you will find a list of reasons people commonly say that it works for them. You can use this to understand why your child uses self-injury to feel better.

Biological Contributors

Much remains unknown about the genetic and biological influences on self-injury behaviors. What we do know comes from several important types of studies, such as examinations of twin studies, which are large databases containing information on hundreds or thousands of pairs of twins. Such studies permit a deeper understanding of the relative contributions of both the genetic and environmental factors that increase risk for self-harm. Information also comes from studies of extreme environmental deprivation and how this alters the ways in which individuals interact with the world. And, finally, we can learn from studies of the neurobiology of self-injury and how it may serve as a pain reliever for the brain. All of these will be discussed in turn, in order to provide a better understanding of what scientists know so far.

How Do Nature and Nurture Intersect?

How much of our behavior is driven by nature versus nurture? In other words, do your genes or your environment influence how you develop and what you become? This has been a topic of discussion in scientific circles for hundreds of years. Since the late 1800s, scientists such as Sir Francis Galton have demonstrated how the study of twins provides a unique understanding of the complex interaction of genes and environment in shaping individual behavior and life trajectories. Classic twin study experimental design is based on comparing identical twins (who share all of their genes) with fraternal twins (who share roughly 50% of their genes). The assumption is that because each twin pair is raised in roughly the same environment, any additional similarities found between identical twins above and beyond what is found in fraternal twins can be ascribed

> We now know that most behaviors and characteristics are a combination of genes and environment, but exploration continues on how these two forces intersect.

to genetic rather than environmental forces. Of course, we now know that most behaviors and characteristics are a combination of genes and environment, but exploration continues on how these two forces intersect.

Research has consistently found that parental experience with self-injury and suicidal thoughts and behaviors is a risk factor for adolescent self-injury and suicidal thoughts and behaviors.[8] However, how much of this risk for self-harm or suicide is due to genes that are passed from one generation to the next? Or, perhaps it is environmental influences that play the critical role in transmitting self-harm behaviors, things like common social forces acting on the family, like persistent poverty or drug abuse? In a recent study of more than 6,000 twin pairs from the Netherlands Twin Registry, researchers found that, among men, genes and environment equally influenced development of risk for self-injury and suicidal behaviors. In women, while both factors contributed, genetics appeared to play a greater role than environment in the development of self-injury.[9] While analysis of twins is one strategy that scientists have for gaining insight into the contributions of genes and environment, this type of work is limited in what it can teach us about *how* the environment contributes to an individual's ability to survive or thrive.

Sometimes scientific knowledge is gained from natural occurrences taking place around the world. Environmental "extremes" that illustrate ideal conditions or extreme deprivation are useful for gaining a better understanding of how the environment can dramatically affect growth and healthy development. Research of this type was conducted in the 1990s on institutionalized, orphaned Romanian infants who had spent months, sometimes years, in extreme emotional deprivation. This occurred as a by-product of political policies and difficult economic conditions in Romania that led to a large number of unwanted or uncared for children. Once these conditions were discovered and the majority of infants and children were placed in foster and adoptive homes, scientists were able to observe how much change, or "plasticity," was possible in development as a result of radically different environmental conditions.

What they saw was shocking. Upon adoption, many of the children were able to make rapid developmental gains over a period of several years. However, nearly a third of children adopted after the age of 6 months experienced continued difficulties in social functioning. They expressed autistic-like qualities and difficulties forming attachments.[10] Regardless of what was for all intents and purposes an improved environment, these children were not able to progress in their normal development. This helped researchers gain understanding of the complex interactions between genetic predisposition, timing of experiences, and extreme environmental conditions. In the case of the Romanian orphans older than 6 months, regardless of their improved living situations upon adoption, the experience of extreme emotional deprivation during early development effectively stunted emotional growth for a large portion of them (but not all).

What does this have to do with self-injury? As a result of studies like these, we now know that the life experiences we have (environmental factors such as abuse, neglect, poverty, parental alcohol abuse) may lead to a series of genetic alterations. Termed an "epigenetic cascade," this involves a complex series of genetic alterations caused by difficult environmental factors that contribute to some of the inheritance of disease and disease risk. This includes predisposition to suicidality and/or other self-harming behaviors.[11] We think of this as similar to the formation of a mighty river, with multiple smaller streams feeding into this river, adding to the size and character of the river. In other words, genetics are not just what you are "born with," but are also something that evolves and changes in subtle ways over time based on contributions of environment and experiences.[12]

These studies contribute a lot to understanding the bigger *Why* of why a particular person may or may not be predisposed to self-injury. But we must also look to the inner landscape each of us holds in order to understand the smaller *why* of any given self-injury episode. For that, we need to understand the role of key neurotransmitters, or messengers within the brain, which most self-injury scholars believe are linked to the development and maintenance of self-injury.

The Neurobiology of Self-Injury

With the advent of brain imaging technology, our ability to understand self-injurious behavior from a biological perspective has dramatically improved. While we have much to learn about how impulses originate and become habitual and how biology contributes to why some people self-injure and others do not, we know that many of the psychiatric conditions associated with self-injury, such as depression, bipolar disorder, and borderline personality disorder, share involvement of the same neurotransmitters.

There are many different types of neurotransmitters, and they each have different functions and associated states of consciousness or feelings. By moving in and out of different brain regions, they tell the body what it feels (for instance, cold, hot, hungry, tired) and what it needs to do to come into equilibrium (eat, find warmth, rest). For example, temporary spikes in levels of adrenalin, a neurotransmitter with which many of us are familiar, cause most people to feel pumped up, energetic, or ready to respond to a challenging environment. The interactions between neurotransmitters, what else is going on in the body (such as sleep deprivation), and how we are engaged with our environment (such as the experience of extreme stress) can be complex. However, it is increasingly clear that imbalances in key neurotransmitters *over time* contribute to adverse physical and mental health conditions like self-injury.

> It is increasingly clear that imbalances in key neurotransmitters *over time* contribute to adverse physical and mental health conditions like self-injury.

One of the key collections of neurotransmitters to which self-injury is linked is the opioid family. *Endogenous* (meaning they are created naturally in the body) opioids are responsible for controlling pain, slowing breathing, and producing a generally calming effect on mood. Opioid derivatives, like morphine or heroin (obviously not created naturally in the body), form the base of many prescription pain medications, such as OxyContin or codeine. The "homeostasis model" of self-injury suggests that levels of these naturally occurring opioids and what are known as *opioid receptors* in the brain tend to be lower among adolescents who engage in self-injury as compared with individuals who do not engage in self-injury.[11] In other words, individuals may use self-injury to induce the brain to release these endogenous opioids, which is experienced by the body as relief in times of stress. This is consistent with how teens talk about their self-injury, saying that they injure in order to "feel something, even if pain" or to "relieve feeling 'numb' or empty."

Serotonin is a neurotransmitter responsible for helping to regulate many factors that contribute to an individual's overall sense of well-being, such as mood, sleep, appetite, learning, memory, and im-pulsiveness. Serotonin has also been implicated in the development and maintenance of self-injury. Several studies of adolescents have found lower levels of serotonin among individuals who self-injure, suggesting that people who self-injure are uniquely vulnerable to negative mood states and mood swings, as well as impulsiveness, all of which are strong contributors to the desire to self-injure.[13] In this case, the serotonin released as a result of self-injury may tem-porarily elevate mood. Indirect support for the role of serotonin in self-injury comes also from the benefit that some individuals gain from using selective-serotonin reuptake inhibitors (SSRIs), which allow for more serotonin to be available in the brain and can help to reduce depression levels and impulsivity among individuals who self-injure. It is important to note that while SSRIs such as fluox-etine (Prozac), sertraline (Zoloft), paroxetine (Paxil), citalopram (Celexa), and escitalopram (Lexapro) have been found to be effective in treating clinical depression in adults, controversy exists around the use of these in children and adolescents.

How does one end up with low levels of these key neurotransmitters? The science on this is less clear. It is possible that early (even in utero) or chronic abuse, trauma, or neglect can interfere with key brain and central nervous system development processes that translate into lower levels of the neurotransmitters responsible for healthy self-regulation. Our interactions can affect these systems. Individuals who exercise regularly, for example, can increase levels of circulating endogenous opioids, creating a sense of calm and contentment both during exercise and long afterward. In fact, as mentioned earlier, those who self-injure report that exercise reduces their urges to self-injure. Regular meditation and other stress-relieving behaviors have a similar effect. Likewise, chronic engagement in some behaviors (like sitting for long hours, eating poorly, avoiding work, ruminating) have a depressive effect on these "feel good" neurotransmitters. Because of this, understanding what causes what is critical.

What is clear is that our particular biochemistries, at any moment, are a result of a complex interaction between biology and our external environments, a veritable "cascade" of mutually reinforcing effects. For instance, lower serotonin levels in multiple family members, perhaps as a result of a shared genetic predisposition, are associated with a greater degree of family conflict and negative interaction.

Understanding how these biological tendencies operate in individuals and within families, and how these may contribute to shaping family dynamics, provides more options for families hoping to make some positive changes.[14]

Science Spotlight: Physical Activity, Mood, and Self-Injury

In 2007, Matthew Wallenstein and Matthew Nock published a case study of a 26-year-old woman with a lengthy history of NSSI on average a couple of times per week.[15] In addition to the twice weekly counseling she received, the patient was encouraged to exercise three times a week for 1 hour over 5 weeks using a workout video provided and to also exercise whenever she had an urge to self-injure. She was asked to record her feelings and any self-injury urges and behaviors each day. The results were promising, with the frequency of self-injury decreasing significantly. Furthermore, her mood improved each time that she exercised, and her urges to self-injure were also significantly reduced following every single bout of exercise. Of note, the patient stopped exercising at one time point during the course of the study. During this time of no exercise, she began again engaging in self-injury regularly. Once she began to exercise again, no episodes of self-injury were reported for the remaining weeks of the study. Eight weeks later, the patient reported continued improvements to both her mental and physical health.

This should come as no surprise to many of us who regularly exercise. Physical activity is a mood booster, associated with an increase in enthusiasm and energy.[16] Research over the past 5 years provides encouraging support for using physical activity to improve mood and prevent depressive symptoms in adolescents and adults.[17,18] This is particularly important given that the transition from adolescence into young adulthood is often associated with increases in depressive symptoms. In a large study following youth from aged 15–21, those teens who engaged in greater amounts of physical activity at age 15 were less likely to develop depressive symptoms and experienced less depression throughout their teen years into young adulthood.[19]

Aerobic forms of physical exercise have been shown to regulate mood and to stimulate the release of beta-endorphin. This may be particularly important to those who self-injure because self-injury is often done for tension relief, emotional regulation, and management of negative mood states. When our bodies are engaged in physical exercise, they release endogenous opioids, which may also play a key role in the process of emotion regulation. One study asked 39 young adults who self-injure how often and how helpful they found 48 different methods that could be used to cope with urges to self-injure.[20] Two thirds (65.7%) of them reported using sports or recreational exercise to cope with and resist NSSI urges. Of these, 62.5% rated exercise as "very helpful" in managing urges to self-injure on average 85% of the time.

Engaging in physical activity may buffer against depression by fostering a sense of social connection, increasing self-esteem and self-efficacy, and providing a healthy outlet for managing one's emotions. Robert Thayer and colleagues proposed that self-regulation of mood involves managing the two dimensions of energy and tension to their optimal levels.[21] From this perspective, most of us have strategies that we use to regulate these two dimensions, such as using nicotine, alcohol, or other substances; consuming sugar or caffeine; and exercise. According to Thayer's theory, moderate exercise is one of the most effective mood-regulating behaviors as it both enhances energy levels and reduces tension levels.

The US Department of Health and Human Services recommends teenagers have 60 minutes or more of physical activity each day.[22] This can involve structured activities, such as team sports, or unstructured activities, such as walks in nature. Furthermore, physical activity can be engaged in all at once or in small bouts of 2–10 minutes—as long as it adds up to 60 minutes per day, both physical and mental health benefit.[23]

Pain Offset Relief Theory: A Biological Explanation of Why Self-Injury Makes People Feel Better

Another important biological component has to do with the way pain is experienced among those who self-injure. It is common to assume that individuals who self-injure experience pain differently from those who do not or perhaps that they do not experience pain at all. After all, why is it that so many people report that self-injury both reduces bad feelings and leads to good feelings?

Early research on this question showed that, regardless of the type of pain experienced (such as pain felt from cold, heat, or pressure), people who engage in self-injury *do* tend to tolerate physical pain for longer periods than do other people. This led to questions about whether the pain they experienced actually hurt them less or whether they simply tolerated it differently. It also led to questions about why *increasing* physical pain on the body would help to *reduce* their experience of emotional pain.

Research in these areas has yielded some interesting and important findings that relate the experience of physical pain and emotional pain. Joseph Franklin, Nancy Eisenberg, and other pioneers in this area have shown that *physical pain itself does not make people feel emotionally better, but something about the offset, or removal, of physical pain does.* In other words, the sense of relief that happens after you remove a painful stimulus—such as removing your finger from a hot pan, finishing a difficult exercise routine, or feeling invigorated after getting off a terrifying roller coaster—is one of the basic human pain experience processes used by individuals who self-injure. *Pain offset theory* suggests that the relief from physical pain that follows a self-injury event essentially tricks the brain into perceiving relief of emotional pain, too.[24]

> *Pain offset theory* suggests that the relief from physical pain that follows a self-injury event essentially tricks the brain into perceiving relief of emotional pain, too.

How does this work? Early brain researchers assumed that we would find specific areas in the brain responsible for specific capacities (such as seeing, hearing, processing emotion, and registering physical pain). This is not true. It turns out that our brains do not have specialized areas for specific (e.g., fear, happiness) or even general (e.g., thoughts, emotion, memory) experiences. Instead, the primary processing area of the brain is involved in many different tasks at the same time, and these tasks may be very different in nature. Moreover, studies find that there is a large degree of "neural overlap" between seemingly very different brain activities. For example, there is a high degree of neural overlap between physical pain and emotional pain (in particular, in areas called the anterior cingulate cortex [ACC] and the anterior insula [AI]). Indeed, research so far suggests that our brains do not strongly distinguish between "feeling hurt" physically and "feeling hurt" emotionally. As a result, the pain-offset studies have led to some odd and fascinating findings. For example, some physical pain medications, such as Tylenol, that target the ACC and AI parts of the brain actually reduce emotional pain as well as physical pain (although probably not as quickly as many of us would like)!

This has interesting implications for self-injury. One of the most common reasons individuals give for injuring themselves is that it reduces emotional pain. If, in fact, brains cannot distinguish well between emotional and physical pain, and if the same brain areas are responsible for sensing and reacting to both, it is not hard to imagine how the brain might "link" the two experiences. And, when it comes to reducing pain, emotional pain is often *much* more difficult for many people to reduce or turn off—it takes skill, experience, and energy. On the other hand, physical pain is very easy to turn off: simply stopping cutting the skin leads to physical pain offset.[15] As one teenager described:

> When the emotions are so strong and no one seems to understand, and it builds up so much that I get a headache, I just feel sick at everything. I feel like the [self-injury] is an escape at that one moment. It's in circumstances like that when I get really intense and just feel like I can't release it any other way.
>
> —*Sarah, 16, on why self-injury works for her*

Add to this the fact that individuals who self-injure are often more sensitive to emotional discomfort *and* they're also often more sensitive to when this physical pain is turned off. When these two are combined, it begins to explain why emotional pain can so effectively be relieved when that physical pain is removed.[25]

This is an important point for several reasons. First, it shows that people who engage in self-injury are not "wired" differently to enjoy pain. Instead, pain offset relief is experienced by nearly all living things, not only those who self-injure. Second, it suggests that self-injury does not simply act as a distraction from bad thoughts and feelings. Sure, there may be some distraction as a result of pain, but pain offset relief appears to both decrease bad feelings and increase good feelings.

What does our understanding of pain offset theory mean for helping people who self-injure? It is possible that this information will assist in the future development of new medications. But there is suggestion that certain therapy techniques may help to alter the connection between these neural processes of emotional and physical pain. For example, a recent study provided people who self-injure with brief cognitive therapy to improve their self-worth. It turns out that developing better self-worth led to being able to endure a much *shorter* period of physical pain. In other words, participants were less likely to want to endure pain when they were feeling better about themselves. These findings offer insights into what are likely to be effective therapeutic strategies.

Psychological Contributors

A psychological approach to understanding self-injury helps us to understand the emotions, thoughts, and behaviors that lead to and maintain self-injury. It typically involves what's commonly termed a "behavioral approach." A behavioral approach pays particular attention to the antecedents and consequences, or the "proximal" or closest factors occurring both before and after a particular behavior or situation. For instance, in the case of Arnold, a fifth-grader who resists doing his homework in the evening, a behavioral approach would aim to learn more about what events are leading up to homework time (e.g., Arnold is just home from school and is tired and hungry; or, Arnold's older brother and sister are distracting him by playing video games in the same room) and what is occurring as a result of his not completing his homework (e.g., Arnold's mom throws her hands up in the air and says she gives up; Arnold is sent to his room for "time-out," where he watches his favorite TV show). As you might imagine, how you manage the situation with Arnold will vary depending on what specific events take place before and after Arnold's homework refusals.

In the case of self-injury, it takes careful consideration of the events leading up to the self-injury: What events cause the desire to injure? When does it usually happen? What forms of self-injury are used? What areas of the body are affected? It's also important to discern what happens in the immediate aftermath and later following the event: How do family members respond to the injury? What sort of emotional relief is obtained? Often, the particularities noted are not visible to the eye but instead involve the thoughts, perceptions, and emotions experienced by an individual. Each of these pieces of information offer clues about the reasons behind how and why self-injury works. This kind of information can also provide helpful insight into the meaning of the act, where it fits into the larger story of one's life, and where there may be opportunities to offer new ways of thinking about or handling the situations that give rise to the behavior. Unfortunately, it is often far easier to identify important contributors that led to an episode of self-injury *after the fact* than it is to predict self-injury before it occurs.

Most commonly, individuals who self-injure use psychological and emotional words to describe "why" they do it. Siang, for example, described it like this:

> I guess it's like you do it so you feel control. Then you act more confident because of it. Then that leads you to really believe that you're in control, and you're badass or tough or confident. It is like a self-fulfilling prophecy. . . . I remember hitting the walls in my parents house and making holes in them. [What set it off was] just something small. What's weird is just the way I reacted to that tiny thing—I would make a huge deal out of it and just want to hurt myself somehow, but usually [it was] just little arguments, and people would get really surprised that I reacted so violently.
>
> —*Siang, age 20*

The behavioral approach suggests that self-injury occurs because of several primary reasons: to regulate and manage painful inner emotional turmoil, to communicate and express psychological distress, and to refocus one's attention away from painful situations.[26] In these ways, self-injury can be deeply symbolic and very effective at altering perceptions of victimization or feeling out of control and turning this into a sense of calm and containment. Individuals who self-injure often see the self-injury as symbolic—doing physically what they wish they could do emotionally—control the experience from start to finish. Mary described it this way:

> It was like a surge of . . . something. When you're angry or upset you feel like you're burning inside, you know, and you just feel it everywhere. And cutting would focus it, and make it something to deal with, something that I could fix. I think a big part of it was it was so self-contained. Like I alluded to, I always kept all my emotions inside anyway, so that was a way of keeping it within but putting it in a way I could deal with it. Because you cut your arm, you can put Neosporin on it, you can make sure that it's healing and that it's not leaving a mark. You can watch the marks fade . . . if anybody had asked I would have said it was cat scratches. . . . It kind of brought things to the surface in a way that I could deal with, that I could take care of on my own.
>
> —*Mary, age 24, on why self-injury worked for her*

Experiential Avoidance: A Psychological Explanation of Why Self-Injury Makes People Feel Better

The desire to regulate feelings and redirect attention away from feeling powerless and toward feeling powerful is very common. This helps us to better understand how self-injury can become so appealing for some and also how difficult it can be to give up the behavior once it begins.

This desire to avoid or escape strong feelings is called *experiential avoidance.*[27] This model is based on the premise that engaging in self-injury serves to reduce or stop unwanted emotions. Wanting to avoid strong, usually negative (but not always) emotions is part of what is often called the "cycle of shame" or the "distress cycle." This pattern often looks like the one in Figure 4.1.

In brief, this cycle describes the "build-up phase," where an individual experiences some situation or event that is upsetting (such as an argument with a best friend, parent, or romantic partner). This

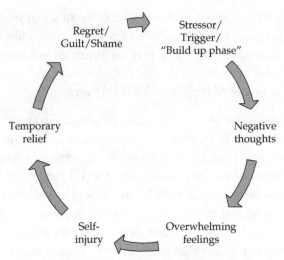

FIGURE 4.1 Experiential avoidance: The cycle of shame.

results in the experience of negative thoughts (e.g., "I'm not loved or appreciated") and strong emotions (anger, shame, sadness, frustration) that can feel as though they may be occurring nearly simultaneously. These feelings then drive a powerful desire to escape from them that culminates in an act of self-injury. The self-injury, for reasons just described, is very effective at reducing the experience of those strong emotions—that is, until the next time. While the self-injury can be effective in the short term, it tends to eventually lead to a sense of shame and/or failure (e.g., "Why can't I control myself?" "Why do I always do this?")—strong feelings that set the stage for the whole process to begin again. Over time, this can become a vicious cycle, with self-injury serving as a short-term safe haven that tends to undermine a long-term sense of self-worth, security, and well-being. Mary described this in our interview:

> **Interviewer:** So in that case probably watching it heal must have felt pretty good, too.
> **Mary:** I was actually really mostly paranoid most of the time when I was watching it heal in that I didn't ever want anybody to know. Every time you do it, you think you're crazy, you know! It's never normal.
> **Interviewer:** So having it felt like evidence that something was wrong.

Mary: Yeah, yeah. So I think that's why I never did it any worse: because I wanted it [the self-injury] to go away. I wanted it to do its job then, at that moment, but then I wanted it to go away.

—Mary, age 24, on the cycle of self-injury

The cycle can also become quite habitual and difficult to stop. James describes it like this:

It was just like every time I got angry or sad, I immediately would cut. And, you know, it [the urge to cut] would get stronger and I would have to do more and more and more damage and deeper cutting, or I was unsatisfied with the whole thing.

—James, age 17, on the cycle of self-injury

So, self-injury can become a coping strategy that works—at least for a while. Creating a space for open conversation with your child about his or her experience of these processes will allow you a clearer window into the emotions and thoughts that drive the urge to injure.

Let's pause a moment to take a closer look at some of the most common patterns noted among self-injurious individuals as a group. While these may not describe your experience in particular, it is likely that you will recognize some of these qualities in your child or loved one.

Emotional Sensitivity

Individuals who self-injure feel emotions more strongly than others and have trouble regulating them. Not surprisingly, studies of adolescents have consistently found that emotion regulation is the most commonly cited reason for self-injury. Teens who self-injure commonly report experiencing strong negative emotions before they self-injure (such as anger, sadness, and anxiety), with these improving during and especially after self-injury. Consistent with what we know about the biology of self-injury and pain offset theory, in general, individuals who self-injure are likely to report experiencing more in-tense emotions, more difficulty identifying their feelings, less skill in managing these emotions, and greater effort avoiding negative emotions altogether than adolescents who have never engaged in self-injury.

Let's see if we can unpack this further. With regard to emotional sensitivity, we know that individuals who self-injure tend to feel deeply. They are more likely to experience more negative than positive emotions, both just before their self-injury episodes as well as in their everyday emotional experiences. For example, a recent study asked individuals who do and do not self-injure to complete a daily diary for 14 days and to rate a list of 20 specific emotions experienced over the course of each day. The individuals who self-injured reported higher levels of negative emotions and lower levels of positive emotions.[28] In other words, those who self-injure appear prone to being self-critical and to experiencing intense self-directed anger and dislike. Whether these emotions and perceptions are what contribute to or are a result of self-injury (or both) is unclear, but it is clear that they are very common once the behavior has become a part of someone's life.

> Those who self-injure appear prone to being self-critical and to experiencing intense self-directed anger and dislike.

With strong negative emotions comes a need to manage them in some way. Here is where self-injury comes in since it offers a quick and easy way to reduce the strong feelings. This form of "emotion regulation" works by allowing someone a quick and effective way to express strong emotions while simultaneously "taking control" of emotions that may be perceived as overwhelming and otherwise unmanageable. Studies consistently show that more than half of the teens and young adults who self-injure report using self-injury "to stop bad feelings." Indeed, not only does self-injury reduce negative feelings, some people report positive feelings in the aftermath as well—usually "calm" and/ or "a sense of relief" from negative emotions. As one teen described, "I had all of this angst, and after I cut I'd feel I could go downstairs and have dinner. I always felt a release."

Thought Suppression as a Way to Avoid Strong Emotions

Despite the struggle with strong emotion, the outward appearances of individuals who injure varies considerably. Many individuals who injure show no outward signs at all of emotional disequilibrium and are good at managing public image, even in the throes of inner turmoil. As Wendy Lader, director of Self-Abuse Finally Ends (SAFE) Alternatives,[29] has observed about the individuals coming through her program, "Many are sensitive, perfectionists, and overachievers."

> Yeah, I always could shut off anything. I was very good at compartmentalizing my emotions from a very young age, and just continue functioning regardless of whatever. And in freshman year, my academics were probably part of what saved me because that could take up huge amounts of my time that I didn't have to think about how miserable I was.
>
> —*Lydia, age 23, on her ability to compartmentalize thoughts and feelings*

Evident in Lydia's comment is the idea of "thought suppression," or the deliberate attempt to not think of something painful. Thought suppression is a cognitive strategy aimed at gaining control of negative thoughts and the upsetting emotions that result from these thoughts. In other words, thoughts create unpleasant emotions, which then leads to an attempt to suppress or bury these thoughts. Often, this strategy is unproductive, leading to an even greater focus on those thoughts. It's as if you've been instructed to *not* think of a white bear. Try as you might, the thought of a white bear is likely to creep into your mind. In the case of self-injury, in order to manage increasingly negative thoughts and their resulting emotions, people often revert to self-harm to distract themselves.

Indeed, research supports this relationship. Adolescents with a tendency to suppress unwanted thoughts report engaging in self-injury in order to reduce their experience of uncomfortable emotions. Many report that they were discouraged from expressing emotions, particularly anger and sadness. One study found that, among individuals who self-injure shown a short video clip that was meant to induce sadness, those participants who resisted feeling the sadness were more likely to report an urge to self-injure after viewing the clip than were those who let themselves feel sad. Similarly, among teenagers who report experiencing high levels of psychological distress, those who attempt to suppress or bury their upsetting thoughts and emotions often feel (and act on) very strong desires to self-injure.

Difficulty Tolerating Stress and Distress

Research suggests that individuals who self-injure are less able (or less willing) to tolerate stress and distress than their non–self-injuring peers and that they use self-injury as a method of escaping a distressing experience.

> Someone could say something wrong, and I would take it the wrong way, and any kind of little thing would set me off and I would turn to cutting.
>
> —*Sophie, age 19*

Clinicians have long described those who self-injure as having difficulty with tolerating life's naturally occurring highs and lows. Lab-based studies provide support for these findings. In one study, a researcher repeatedly informed each participant that his or her answers on a series of card-sorting tasks were incorrect. Individuals who self-injured were significantly more likely to express frustration and greater physiological arousal during this distressing task than were non-injurers. They were also more likely to give up on the task earlier and to have difficulties solving problems once they were distressed. Interestingly, those individuals with a history of self-injury (but not in the past year) reported greater ability to tolerate their emotions and better impulse control than individuals who were still self-injuring.[29] This is important because it offers hope that accepting and tolerating difficult feelings is a skill that can be developed to help stop the self-injury cycle.

Social Contributors

Social models of self-injury view it as a behavior that is undertaken to seek out social connection or attention. In other words, engaging in self-injury serves as a coping strategy that helps to either gain control over or escape from perceived social demands. When people describe the "why" of self-injury as "to try and get a reaction from someone, even if it's negative" and "to get control of a situation," they are describing the social dimension of self-injury. Several specific motivations may be at play, including a desire to communicate distress to others, a desire for connection, or the desire to avoid unwanted social situations. It is important to note, however, that self-injury is rarely undertaken for merely theatrical purposes or group membership ("trying to fit in"). To dismiss self-injury as just attention-seeking or simply as a way to belong negates the need for developing healthy communication and emotion regulation skills.

> To dismiss self-injury as merely attention-seeking or simply as a way to belong negates the need for developing healthy communication and emotion regulation skills.

Communicating Distress or the Desire to Connect

Although we know that it is most common for individuals with regular (even if intermittent) self-injury to report injuring as a means of regulating negative emotion, approximately 15–30% of adolescents and young adults identify social reasons for doing it, usually as a bid for communicating pain or hurt or to convey a desire for connection. Applied to self-injury, the *social signaling hypothesis* suggests that self-injury helps to facilitate social communication as a "high-intensity" behavior. That is, if it could speak, it would be a yell rather than a whisper. In social communication terms, this means that it is more likely to command attention than something more subtle, such as hanging around hoping someone will notice or making an indirect verbal request. For example, Maria said that part of the reason she cut herself in places she knew people might see was a conscious effort to gain her father's attention:

> I wanted him to notice I was suffering. I wanted him to ask me what was wrong; that's what I wanted, I really wanted him to ask me "why?"
>
> —*Maria, age 24*

In this way, Maria's self-injury was intended to communicate, "I hurt and I really want you to notice and do something." Her father, baffled at the behavior and uncomfortable with the feelings it raised, dismissed it as manipulative and remained silent. When used to garner attention in this particular way, it generally does feel manipulative to onlookers. A closer look at cases like this, however, suggests that the driving force is less about a desire to manipulate than about the deep and often childlike desire for *connection* coupled with an inability to ask for this connection in a more direct way. In this case,

Maria was using her behavior to "speak," but her father did not understand the message, so both remained alienated from each other. It is important to note that this is not always the case.

It is true that self-injury can and often does lead to more parental attention in ways that are desired—and sometimes not desired—by the young person. If parents recognize this desire for connection, it is most helpful if they can honor it by creating more authentic, healthy, and sustainable lines of communication. Section 3 of this book offers suggestions on how to develop a deeper connection with your teen.

Avoiding Unwanted Social Situations

Individuals who self-injure sometimes do so in order to avoid unwanted social situations, to avoid doing something unpleasant, or to avoid being with certain people. In this case, self-injury is used to distract self and others from whatever uncomfortable thing is going on or looming in the near future. Common examples of this include stopping parents from fighting or stopping a boyfriend or girlfriend from leaving. In this way, self-injury may be a way to maintain some degree of homeostasis and also divert attention from other forms of life dysfunction (i.e., familial, environmental, or societal). For example, one adolescent we worked with used self-injury to avoid unwanted sexual advances. Her cutting was viewed with disgust and outrage, and so she was able to avoid being further targeted.

Social Contagion

Like germs, behaviors and even emotions and simple thoughts are "contagious" and can spread from one person to another. Social contagion, or the transmission of feelings, attitudes, beliefs, and behavior across groups, has been documented in eating disorders, drug use, suicidal thoughts and behaviors, laughter, exercise, weight gain, and even happiness and depression. While it's not completely clear how this happens, both research and anecdotal study suggest that self-injury can and sometimes does "spread" among youth (and adults). Social contagion episodes have been reported among adolescents and adults living in treatment settings, group homes, prison, and juvenile detention facilities. Anecdotal reports also suggest that self-injury contagion occurs in schools, universities, and community settings.[30] Moreover, the spread of self-injury does not only occur among those who know each other. Widespread introduction and spread of self-injury in mainstream media as well as in virtual and social media venues has led to contagion.[31]

> Both research and anecdotal study suggest that self-injury can and sometimes does "spread" among youth.

But, also like germs, not everybody exposed to self-injury is likely to "catch" it.[32] The factors that make someone vulnerable to self-injury if exposed are (1) a desire to be associated with or fit in with a high-status peer or group in which self-injury is applauded (e.g., Goth or "emo" group affiliation is common in this way), (2) having a close friend who self-injures, (3) age (middle and young high school students are most influenced by their peers and hence more likely to adopt the behavior), and (4) identification with the underlying narratives (life or situation stories) or feelings associated with self-injury (as encountered through a book, web-based community, movie, admired celebrity or musician). With self-injury so much more a part of mainstream culture now, the opportunity for exposure and adoption of the behavior is much higher than it was when it was well-hidden and/or less prevalent.

Activities

Activity 1: Tracking Triggers and the Immediate Consequences of Self-Injury Using the ABC's

Here, you will find a simple log for tracking the Antecedents, Behaviors, and Consequences—the ABC's—of self-injury. We'll devote more time to this in Section 2 of the book, but, for now, we would like you to begin to explore what works best for you in terms of noticing and documenting the ABC's of self-injury. For some, this may involve keeping a journal to record your thoughts and perspectives on the triggers and immediate aftermath of your child's self-injury episodes. For others, it may be helpful to track this information in table format. We've provided a brief outline of such a table here, with an example included. Both caretakers and individuals who injure can do this activity; it can be helpful to compare notes.

Tracking the ABC's of Self-Injury (Sample)

Date/Time	Antecedent	Behavior	Consequences
	What happened immediately before the self-injury?	What self-injury thoughts or behavior(s) took place?	What happened immediately after the self-injury?
3/21, 3:30 pm	My child came home from school clearly upset about something that had happened.	She went to her room and refused to open the door when I asked her if we could talk. I was terrified that she was going to harm herself.	She refused to talk to me for several hours. I was anxious, but also angry and felt guilty for feeling angry with her.

Tracking the ABC's of Self-Injury

Date/Time	Antecedent	Behavior	Consequences
	What happened immediately before the self-injury?	What self-injury thoughts or behavior(s) took place?	What happened immediately after the self-injury?

Activity 2: Reflection Activity

Self-reflection can be an important part of the journey that you will make with your teen over the coming months and years as you work through struggles and build on strengths. Your intentions and goals will likely change over time depending on your needs and your teen's, but we hope this is the beginning of a productive process that offers you insight into your teen's self-injury and the factors that might help to explain *Why*.

As you review what we have learned about the *Why* of self-injury, consider the following questions. Feel free to write down your intentions or goals relating to these.

1. How can I learn from this? How does this help me understand my child's particular story?

2. How might our family environment or dynamic be contributing to the persistence of self-injury?

3. How does our family environment or dynamic encourage and support change and growth? What goals can I work toward?

4. What can I do to improve communication between my child and myself?

5. What can I do to be more supportive and nonreactive to my child's struggles with self-injury? How can I provide structure while balancing her or his need for independence?

6. And, perhaps most importantly, how can I integrate this information into my life and move forward, personally and in unison with my child, in spite of the challenge self-injury has posed for us all?

Activity 3: How Does It Help? Reasons for Self-Injury

Here is a list of reasons that someone might engage in self-injury. As we have discussed, some of these are more common than others. For this activity, we would like you to review the list and consider how your child might be using self-injury. Then, if your child is willing to have a conversation with you about this, check out your assumptions with him or her. This will allow you to learn more about how self-injury is helping your child, and it might give you insights into how you might be able to better support him or her in the effort to stop injuring.

1. To avoid school, work, or other activities
2. To relieve feeling "numb" or empty
3. To get attention
4. To feel something, even if it was pain
5. To avoid having to do something unpleasant you don't want to do
6. To get control of a situation
7. To try to get a reaction from someone, even if it's a negative reaction
8. To receive more attention from your parents or friends
9. To avoid being with people
10. To punish yourself
11. To get other people to act differently or change
12. To be like someone you respect
13. To avoid punishment or paying the consequences
14. To stop bad feelings
15. To let others know how desperate you were
16. To feel more a part of a group
17. To get your parents to understand or notice you
18. To give yourself something to do when alone
19. To give yourself something to do when with others
20. To get help
21. To make others angry
22. To feel relaxed

Taken from the Functional Assessment of Self-Mutilation (FASM), a self-injury assessment developed by Dr. Lloyd-Richardson and colleagues and originally cited in Lloyd-Richardson, E. E., Perrine, N., Dierker, L., & Kelley, M. L. (2007). Characteristics of non-suicidal self-injury in a community sample of adolescents. *Psychological Medicine*, 37(8), 1183–1192.[32]

Section 2

Recovery, Treatment, and Growth

Ending Self-Injury

I really looked at myself and told myself "I'm better than that."
—Cecilia, 22, on why she stopped self-injuring

Why and How People Stop Self-Injury

By now, you're probably aware that, for many people, self-injury is typically not something that goes away quickly. For individuals who rely on it often or who use it to meet a variety of needs, the pattern usually takes time to change. This is because healing is about more than just stopping the act of injury—it requires complex changes in the relationships among thoughts, emotions, and behavior. Because the process of thoughts leading to emotions and actions can happen very quickly, it will take some time to "unpack" the process enough for change to happen. Indeed, many of the important things that need to happen first involve subtle shifts in thinking about what self-injury is doing and, in particular, why it works. These shifts lead to subtle but cumulative changes in feelings and eventually to changes in behavior, although these changes may not be visible to others for quite a while (we'll discuss the relationships among thoughts, feelings, and behavior in more detail in Chapter 9).

It is rare that someone who has stopped self-injuring can say exactly how it happened. It may not be until much later that the key change moments or factors are visible. In our studies of why people stop self-injury, we find three broad categories: changes in connections with others, better emotion regulation capacity, and fear of consequences.[1] Here are examples of the kinds of statements we encountered in this study. When you read these, notice that the majority of changes cited reflect changes in *thoughts and feelings*:

- *Positive connections with others*: "I entered into a loving relationship."
  "Some of my high school friends were really concerned about what they knew, and talking to them helped a lot."
- *Negative effect on loved others*: "I stopped because of the people that loved me at the time. I wasn't just hurting myself, but I was hurting the people that cared about me. That was hard for me to understand, but once it clicked, I was done."
- *Removal of negative relationships*: "Space away from family/ frustration."
- *Professional/therapeutic support*: "Through the program of recovery that I follow for my substance abuse problem (AA) and through the assistance of my therapist/psychiatrist, I have learned that I am not alone in those feelings and have been shown real solutions for the uncomfortable feelings I have."
- *Enhanced self-awareness*: "I also developed more of a sense of proportion: by which I mean, firstly, that I started to realize that however bad I feel, it's probable that I'll feel better at some point in future, and that I should not act in ways that might permanently diminish my happiness; and secondly, that my emotional distress is minor in comparison to that of many other people."
- *Coping skills (tools/behaviors or direct differences)*: "I realized I could cope with my emotions in less destructive ways. I practice martial arts and work out to focus my mind, being able to spar with someone else helps, too."
- *Life circumstances changed*: "I am happy with my life now, there is no reason for me to be nervous or scared or angry all the time."

- *Maturity*: "I grew out of it and realized I didn't need attention that badly."
  "Most of it I attribute to maturing, to growing out of the raging hormones of adolescence."
- *Fear of consequences*: "I cut too deeply and scared myself."
  "I don't want to have scars; they're ugly."

These kinds of reflections are pretty common, but they gloss over the work it can take to make significant change. On the surface, these reasons seem straightforward and logical. It can seem as though simply deciding one day that self-injury is not a good way to deal with stress and that it is time to "grow up" translates immediately into discontinuation of the behavior. As if it were that easy! For some people struggling with self-injury, this may be true—particularly if it is not something used regularly. For more habitual self-injury users, there are likely to be many small moments that build up to revelations like these before cessation happens. In other words, ending self-injury is not a decision as much as it is a continuous set of decisions and many stitched-together moments of facing hard feelings, memories, or experiences.

When combined with trying out new perspectives, reactions, and skills, it can all feel pretty risky, even when it leads to positive outcomes. It can feel really good to experience new breakthroughs and patterns or to allow oneself to feel deep sadness, fear, anger, or vulnerability without acting on one's body (or on someone else). But these feelings and new experiences can also be scary or even terrifying. This may be particularly true for people who have learned that guarding emotions is the only way to feel safe or for those who fear that these good feelings will eventually end and that they will be left feeling bad again. For these reasons, it can be helpful for loved ones and other supporters, like you, to understand what goes into the healing process and how to help support it.

The Healing Process

What I like most is seeing the changes in her as she has grown in self-awareness and understanding. Seeing how she is able to accept herself now. Seeing those things translate into a much more socially outgoing child who has developed very close loving relationships with friends and family.

—Ananda, parent of a young adult with a long self-injury history
describing the signs of recovery she observed

One of the most amazing things about being human is our capacity to adapt—often without consciously knowing it. Adapting has helped humans to live in physically challenging environments, to learn from our mistakes, and to cooperate with others. All of these are instrumental for our survival as a species. Every one of us has experienced adaptation. Whether the changes we face are internal or external, we learn to respond, adjust, and (re)establish our own sense of equilibrium over time. This is true whether we are adapting to avoid something we find unpleasant or to add more of something we find pleasant. Think about the last time you went on a vacation: a different daily routine and itinerary forced you to adapt to your surroundings in order to feel comfortable and to make the most of your time away from home. We do something similar with each new addition or challenge that comes into our lives, even if it is not a change in our material environment but, instead, comes in the form of a new emotion or narrative.

What we do not often realize is that adaptation may be large and clearly recognizable, like leaving a bad relationship or making a much-needed job change, or it may be more subtle. It can also start out as an obvious accommodation and then become the "new normal." Think about what happens to a hip joint if someone repeatedly favors one foot because the other is injured and does not heal well. Even though the favoring can become habitual and seem minor, these physical adaptations affect the entire system in ways that compromise our ability to walk correctly over time. In this case, those compensatory movements may result in joint and/or nerve inflammation and soft tissue erosion over time that severely hamper walking ability or require extensive surgery.

> All of us, to some degree, learn to "live with" emotional wounds or sore spots.

The same thing happens emotionally. All of us, to some degree, learn to "live with" emotional wounds or sore spots. Unlike favoring an ankle, though, much of the psychological accommodation process is invisible, even to ourselves. While we may show traces on the outside by subtly (or not so subtly) avoiding certain topics or people, the bigger issue is what happens inside when we do the same thing—avoid or distance ourselves from feelings, thoughts, and/or people or circumstances. These kinds of adjustments can become habitual and psychologically inflammatory, just as they can physically. They can also lead to even more emotional "sore spots" and can become linked to other emotional wounds in ways that ultimately limit healthy functioning. This kind of accumulated emotional stress or avoidance pattern can leave someone feeling like he or she is living in a very small space with no way out. Even worse, when somebody does this for a long time, this very small space can feel very normal and even comforting. She or he can completely fail to grasp the idea that there is a much, much bigger space available if she or he is willing to step into it. Feeling severely depressed, anxious, hopeless, or even suicidal can result from living this way.

Self-injury is often a response to this type of inner environment. With the physical pain of self-injury comes relief from unwanted thoughts, feelings, and/or chronic inner gloom. Unfortunately, the many inner adjustments that have been made in hopes of avoiding or reducing unwanted thoughts and emotions over time are what also contribute to and reinforce this cycle of self-injury and, ultimately, heighten suffering. Learning to live without turning to self-injury (or other negative self-soothing behaviors, such as substance abuse and addictions) takes more than just learning new behavioral habits and coping mechanisms, although that is part of it.

One of the most common reasons for not wanting to stop self-injury is the fear of having no alternative coping strategy: "What am I going to do next time I feel overwhelmed?? I can't just sit with it and do nothing!" This means that learning how not to self-injure requires learning how to deal with strong, unwanted feelings and thoughts in other ways, often ways that at first feel much less effective than self-injury. The important thing to remember is that the reasons that a person begins self-injuring are complex and so, too, is the process of stopping the behavior. Understanding the process of change will allow you to recognize the stages of change in its many forms, support your loved one, and, we hope, stay hopeful along the way.

Stages of Behavior Change

In general, the longer one has engaged in a behavior and the more of a "go-to" behavior it is in times of stress, the more difficult it will be to stop. There are typically stages one goes through in the process of *deciding* to stop and then actually taking steps to make this happen. Although the stages of change idea is largely intuitive, keep in mind that change is a process, that it takes time, and that it can feel scary (even when the benefits are so clear). Figure 5.1 is a general graphical representation of change based on extensive research.[2,3]

There are two important things to note about this model. The first thing you'll likely notice are the stages listed, which describe the common phases of behavior change. We'll talk about each of these later. The other important feature of this model is its spiral shape. Rather than one stage directly leading to the next, as in a direct line of progress, the spiral shape indicates that changing negative behavior is

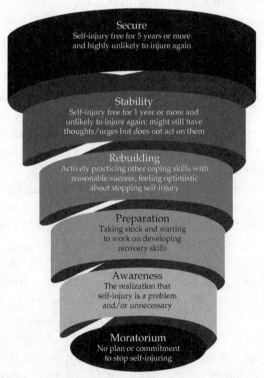

Secure
Self-injury free for 5 years or more and highly unlikely to injure again

Stability
Self-injury free for 1 year or more and unlikely to injure again; might still have thoughts/urges but does not act on them

Rebuilding
Actively practicing other coping skills with reasonable success; feeling optimistic about stopping self-injury

Preparation
Taking stock and starting to work on developing recovery skills

Awareness
The realization that self-injury is a problem and/or unnecessary

Moratorium
No plan or commitment to stop self-injuring

FIGURE 5.1 Stages of change and growth.

really more of a gradual process than it is a linear, step-by-step process. Change can be characterized by small changes, big leaps, and/or feeling as though one is slipping backward for short or longer periods of time. Anyone who has ever tried to lose weight can likely relate to this cycle of progress and slips. However, before we talk more about the way this works, let's talk about the general stages that must be navigated, in some form or another, in order for full healing to happen.

Moratorium

The first stage of change is commonly called Moratorium. Contrary to what it sounds like, a person in this stage does not show or have any interest in stopping his behavior. A person in the Moratorium stage would rather continue in a state of "un-change." He is not likely to recognize the negative impact of self-injury in his life and may describe it as having no negative impact at all (and maybe even a positive one). In general, stopping self-injury is not considered an option for people in Moratorium, and trying to convince them otherwise is typically unfruitful. In this stage, any discussion of change will likely be met with resistance—a literal or symbolic shoulder shrug. Considering a life without self-injury is simply not on the agenda.

Because of the nature of this stage, it can be difficult to actively promote or support self-injury cessation. The expression, "You can lead a horse to water, but you can't make him drink" applies here. You can offer encouragement and opportunity, but you can't force it if someone is not ready to make meaningful change.

> Actively showing appreciation for the ways in which your child shows effort or progress, even if small, helps to positively reinforce constructive steps.

Parents looking for something proactive to do during this stage do have some options. Actively showing appreciation for the ways in which your child shows effort or progress, even if small, helps to positively reinforce constructive steps. Creating opportunities for authentic connection and/or a sense of mastery can also be helpful. While directly confronting the self-injury head on or having direct conversations about it may not be very productive, understanding that it is often a bid for connection and/or an expression of inner

---

Box 5.1 The Moratorium Phase

The most helpful things you can do for someone in the Moratorium phase are:

- Avoid trying to convince, cajole, or threaten
- Focus on raising your own awareness about self-injury
- Consider what resources you may need to help yourself and ensure that your support systems are in place
- Look for and reinforce even minor shifts in your child's awareness, hope, confidence, or intentions (e.g., "You seemed a little more upbeat this week. What went well for you this week?")

---

emotional turmoil can open doors to ideas for helping in these areas. Even if you find your child difficult to be around, increasing opportunities to spend time together doing either fun or productive activities, like learning a new skill together, being present for activities your child is involved in, or just going for ice cream or to see a movie together, can be helpful (Box 5.1).

Supporting opportunities for your child to be engaged in activities, groups, or initiatives outside your home that are in alignment with your child's fundamental interests can also be helpful. Self-injury can signal a low sense of self-esteem or confidence. Supporting opportunities for engagement, especially those that don't feel like a chore to your child, can help her develop some of the inner muscles she's going to need to leave it behind and to engage in more productive activities. And, it's important for parents to look for ways to support things that are of natural interest to their children, not that fulfill a parental agenda or script about what "would be good" for their children.

> We sometimes see self-injury in young people who push themselves very hard.

On the other hand, we sometimes see self-injury in young people who push themselves very hard. In these cases, it might be most useful for parents to clearly and consistently state that their children are loved and will be successful in life even if they are not exceptional in all of the areas they push themselves to be successful in.

Kids with a strong drive to be perfect or to be very high achievers can sometimes feel like they are letting their parents down or like they're going to fail in life if they don't satisfy the ideas of achievement they or their parents have of them. These kids need permission to be "average," and they need affirmation and validation that they can and will still have productive and successful lives even if they are not as exceptional as they believe they have to be. It's truly OK—and they need to know this.

It is common for parents and others who feel responsible for a self-injurious person's well-being to have strongly protective feelings—for their loved one *and* for themselves and others in the family affected by the behavior. With a child who is unwilling to consider change or to admit that there is a problem, a parent may experience unique challenges when concern for a self-injuring family member meets head-on with exposing others to the negative patterns and outcomes of self-injury (such as siblings seeing blood in a shared bathroom space). Parents can find themselves immensely frustrated and confused about how to support and protect everyone involved. This is one of the reasons why having solid support for yourself during this phase is so important.

Awareness

In the Awareness stage (Box 5.2), your child will show evidence of becoming aware of how self-injury is affecting her life, though she may still actively use self-injury to cope. She may acknowledge that self-injury is interfering in various aspects of her life and may also see that it is affecting people closest to her, including parents and friends. This is the stage in which she may begin to cultivate hope for a life free of self-injury. It is important to note that with this hope and new yearning often comes fear and some glimpse of the scary emotions that have been avoided by using self-injury. For example, if self-injury has been used to control unwanted memories or traumas, awareness that self-injury is causing more problems than it is worth and may need to be stopped can cause someone to feel panic at the prospect of having to confront frightening feelings. If these fears arise, it can send someone back into Moratorium for a bit or stall progress.

Box 5.2 The Awareness Phase

The most helpful things you can do for someone in the Awareness phase are:

- Recognize the hard feelings and thoughts which may arise at times (e.g., "I can imagine how frustrating/ difficult this might be for you at times. Is there anything I can do to help lift some of this weight off your shoulders?")
- Reinforce the hope and confidence you have that she is able to face these uncomfortable feelings and thoughts
- Remind your child that while there are some inner mountains she feels she is facing alone, she does not need to be alone. There are people (including you!) who understand and are there to help when it gets overwhelming (for instance, "I really need you to know that you are not alone. How can we work together to both support your need to figure out your own problems and also help you feel less alone with it all?")

The Awareness stage is often more internal than external—meaning that others may not necessarily know that changes in one's relationship to self-injury are happening because the work of this stage is highly personal. Evidence of this stage may emerge through small comments or subtle shifts in behavior.

While the protective instinct will still be very active when living with someone in this phase of change, it may start to give way to the supporter role as well. In the supporter role, parents and caretakers will begin looking for ways to actively support progress and will worry a little less about making sure nothing terrible happens. Hypervigilance, for example, may start to give way to a fledgling sense of hope and the feeling that your child is ready to begin taking responsibility for his healing. This can free up psychological space to look for ways to support this progress. Typically, these shifts in your child's awareness will eventually lead to a greater desire to change his behavior. Once this happens, your teen may move into the next stage.

Preparation

In the Preparation stage of change, your child will likely begin to recognize the need for change and will begin to develop a sense of confidence that change may be possible. It is often in this stage that visible evidence of the desire for change starts to become evident. This could be demonstrated through comments (e.g., "I tried to stop myself from cutting the other night by calling Anna instead") or through clear efforts at changing behavior (e.g., "Instead of cutting the other night I called Anna and we talked. I didn't feel like I needed to do it after that"). In some cases, of course, your child will tell you, and, in other cases, your child might just notice it herself. Individuals in this stage still have doubts about their ability to stop, but the increased confidence and optimism they feel will generally lead to greater commitment to stopping and more openness to trying out new skills they may have resisted before.

In this stage, awareness begins to turn to more active intentions and behavior change strategies and may lead to asking for help, seeking counseling, and/or experimenting with new practices or coping strategies (such as finding new ways to spend time, a new social group, taking up exercise). Be aware that self-injury is still likely in this stage—though you may begin to see a decrease. You may find relief in stepping more fully into the supporter role and seeing more tangible ways to assist your child. Teetering between protector and supporter, however, can also leave parents feeling a little like they are walking on eggshells since slips are common and fear of triggering a self-injury episode may actually increase as everyone becomes a little more relaxed. While there is not a lot to do to stop this from happening, it may be helpful to know that this is normal.

Rebuilding

Typically, the preparation stage gives way to a much more focused set of efforts we think of as the Rebuilding or "action" stage. In this stage, an individual will demonstrate the understanding that stopping is not just wanting to stop, but is also about taking active, necessary steps to stop. Individuals in this stage will often have made active steps in new directions, perhaps taking up a new hobby, getting involved with a new activity at school, or regularly engaging in therapy. It is typically in this stage when people add new abilities to the hope, confidence, and intentions they have already begun cultivating. People in this stage have started to acquire and use new skills (e.g., new strategies for dealing with stressful thoughts or feelings) and have often had some success using these instead of injuring. Although people in the rebuilding stage are not successful every time, the individual is both more confident and hopeful, allowing these newfound interests and skills to help in more broadly defining who they are. Slips may still happen but are more rare.

This can be a nice phase since it can feel like you are working with your child and not in spite of your child. Thinking about yourself as an ally can also have an impact on the kind of language you use and the way you approach your child's process of change. Seeing that you and your child share goals and that your child is increasingly capable of managing "bumps in the road" may transform the natural parental desire to *fix* into a desire to support and enhance your child's own natural healthy efforts toward growth.

> Seeing that you and your child share goals and that your child is increasingly capable of managing "bumps in the road" may transform the natural parental desire to *fix* into a desire to support and enhance your child's own natural healthy efforts toward growth.

The stages we have just reviewed can last from small periods of time, such as months, or go on for much longer periods of time—years or more. It is highly variable because it is in these stages that all of the "work" of changing one's thoughts, feelings, and behaviors is accomplished—figuring out alternative ways of managing, trying out these new strategies, and perfecting their use during different stressful situations.

Stability

Once someone has been self-injury free for 1 year, she is considered to be in the Stability stage of the process. A person in this stage deeply understands what situations or feelings may trigger self-injury and typically uses healthy ways of coping when feeling triggered. While thoughts of and desires to injure might last for a while (sometimes a long while), the urges and thoughts can be tolerated without giving way to self-injury behavior. It is in this stage that resoluteness—steady and well-grounded intention—is established.

As we mentioned earlier, self-injury can come and go, in fits and starts, so it is not uncommon for somebody to be in the stability stage and then experience a relapse of self-injury. For this reason, the benchmark for full healing, inasmuch as that is wholly possible, is somewhat arbitrary. In our work, we have noticed that if someone makes it 3–5 years without injuring, the chances that they will suffer a major relapse are slim.

Secure

For this reason, we think of the 5-year and beyond stage as the Secure stage. Although thoughts and urges may come through at this stage, they are easy to pass by. Individuals in this stage often have and use a variety of healthy coping mechanisms when stress arises.

Although the stage or spiral model that we depicted earlier is a useful way to visualize the progressive steps of change, in real life, change tends to be a bit messier. Change is often cyclical and tends to happen intermittently. And, it can be slippery—we can seem to be making good progress for a while only to "slip" or regress. All of us have had this experience in life. Think about trying to change the way you eat. Once we become aware of what we're doing that's not healthy, we explore other options and then set some intention to change our eating habits; we may find that we are excellent at it for the first few days, weeks, or even months. Typically, however, a vacation comes up, or the holiday season, or a period of extreme stress, and we "slip" (e.g., extra dessert or wine at a holiday party) or "slide" back to earlier patterns (e.g., a series of more or less intentional slips, such as deciding to "just make it through" the holiday season). The trick to success is to not allow these slips and slides to deeply discourage you and to get back on track as quickly as possible. True, deep, sustained change is very difficult to maintain, but still a goal to have and aspire to.

Why Change Can Be So Hard

Why is changing a behavior that leaves so many wounds (both literal and figurative) so difficult? For the casual onlooker, there appear to be no real benefits of self-harm, only the lasting scars and social stigma. This is quite different from the benefits from a less than healthy activity we can all relate to, like a rich but delicious meal. It smells good, tastes good, and is life-sustaining. We need food to live; we don't need self-injury to live. Simple, right? Not so fast. People come to rely on self-injury because it sustains and feeds a set of psychological processes that *feel* protective. It is not uncommon, for example, for someone who self-injures to talk about it as a "friend" or even a "best friend." In this case, self-injury provides protection from unwanted thoughts and feelings, much as a good friend might help to thwart the cruel words—or fists—of a bully. Self-injury can also be symbolically supportive—it can give "voice" to feelings through the physical marks one can make on the body, much like an artist uses a canvas and color to express an emotion without words. People who self-injure commonly describe it as a physical way to express feelings.

> People come to rely on self-injury because it sustains and feeds a set of psychological processes that *feel* protective. It is not uncommon, for example, for someone who self-injures to talk about it as a "friend" or even a "best friend."

If we understand this, then it is easier to understand how the prospect of stopping self-injury may actually feel very limiting to your child. She may be faced with a dilemma, unconsciously asking herself, "what do I do with all of these unwanted thoughts and feelings?" How does she communicate these raw feelings and emotions, which cannot be conveyed with words, to herself, the world, and significant others?

This dilemma leads to one of the most important things for parents and others to know: stopping self-injury may mean that other messy, uncomfortable, and negative things start. One of the most interesting paradoxes of the healing process is that it rarely looks like healing at all, at least for a while. Self-injury has been used as a cork, plugging up any number of unwanted thoughts and emotions. Once the cork has been removed, all of the stuff it was keeping inside tends to come out—sometimes in messy and undignified ways. It can be even more messy and entrenched if there are other mental health conditions and physiological imbalances involved. This may manifest as:

- Seemingly random irritability or emotional volatility
- Very strong negative emotions, often far out of proportion to the trigger (e.g., rage, intense frustration, grief)
- Use of unhealthy replacement behaviors (e.g., use of drugs, food, or other ways of accomplishing what self-injury accomplished)
- Periods of celebration and success followed by periods of major discouragement and resistance
- Setbacks and "slip-ups" in quitting self-injury

Of course, there are likely to be good days, too, days when moods are stable and/or light and when it is clear that there are important shifts in thought and emotion happening. Allow these days and moments to sustain you. Please know that volatility in mood and behaviors is a common part of the process.

Real change is more than just eliminating the behavior. We have observed that underlying successful change are several fundamental attitudes and abilities, all of which are needed to keep progress going: *Hope, Intention, Confidence, Ability,* and *Resolve.* We call this group of qualities "HICAR." These are not easy to adopt or move into when one feels stuck or ambivalent, but they are critical components of the change process.

For those to whom these traits come easily, it can be hard to understand why it's so difficult for others to cultivate them. Cultivating these requires working on more subtle levels where the thoughts and emotions that give rise to self-injury in the first place are stored. We can think of this as the *psychological architecture* of self-injury—the set of core beliefs, experiences, emotional responses, and filters that allow self-injury to prosper. The psychological architecture underlying self-injury and related behaviors is often deeply buried and takes time to surface, examine, and change. This is especially true when that scaffolding is built on past situations, thoughts, and/or feelings that are difficult to remedy because they are still occurring, are not within one's control, or because acknowledging them brings up a lot of powerful or intimidating feelings. This kind of work is usually very emotionally charged. Because change is virtually always incremental, progress may seem slow.

Helping Change Along

A variety of factors affect how quickly or slowly behavior may change. Studies[4] show that how quickly self-injury ends depends on things such as:

- *Frequency.* The more someone injures, the harder it is to stop, probably because it functions as a regulator of powerful underlying emotions.
- *Number of reasons for injuring.* The more reasons one has for injuring, the harder it is to stop.
- *Number and persistence of other mental health challenges.* Feeling chronically high levels of depression and/or anxiety makes it harder to stop.
- *Presence of other, healthier ways of coping with negative thoughts and emotions,* such as support from friends, a creative outlet, humor, and physical activity. More ways of coping make it easier to stop.
- *Recognizing that it is a problem in life.* Acknowledging the problem makes it easier to stop.
- *Feeling socially supported.* Having support makes it easier to stop.
- *Having a sense of meaning in life and/or having higher levels of life satisfaction.* These qualities make it easier to stop.

Truly moving past self-injury includes learning to understand, embrace, tolerate, and transform difficult feelings. This can be a long process and often takes time and effort. Healing will not happen overnight, even if the behavior stops early on in the process.

Gauging Progress: How Do I Know If Progress Is Happening?

Gauging progress can be difficult, especially when it occurs very slowly or incrementally. Because of this, we suggest that you become skilled at looking for small indicators of larger changes. We've included a checklist at the end of this chapter ("The Nuts and Bolts of Healing: A Checklist for Noticing Improvement") that aims to help you build your awareness of small improvements. In general, there are five categories you will want to become adept at watching:

- Self-injury behavior
- Changes in mood
- Thoughts (as evidenced by spoken or written comments or statements)
- Engagement in activities
- Relationships

Shifts in each of these areas can be overt or subtle, and they can signal progress, no change, or increased challenges. Overt shifts are those you notice and which others are likely to notice as well. But since big and sustained changes in behavior or attitude are usually an accumulation of much smaller shifts, becoming adept at tracking and noticing the smaller shifts can assist in supporting and validating progress, particularly for parents who live with and are attuned to their child's moods and activities. You'll see that this checklist describes a few things to watch out for.

How to Spot Reductions in Self-Injury

Keep in mind that this can be difficult to accurately observe because research shows that parents most often overestimate how much they know about their child's self-injury behavior and underestimate how often it is occurring.[5] Individuals who are actively self-injuring are not very likely to be completely honest on this front because they don't want to disappoint people who love them (and because they may not want to be totally honest with themselves either). In general, relying on what you observe, rather than on what your child tells you in this regard, might be a little more helpful.

Take advantage of opportunities to notice new wounds without prying or being invasive. For example, family outings where a child wears short sleeves or a bathing suit can give you an opportunity to subtly observe a little more thoroughly than is possible when fully clothed. Similarly, going to the gym together, if you're in the same locker room, may also provide an opportunity like this. It is important, however, not to demand a child show you her scars or places on her body where there might be new wounds. If you are in deep need for information about the status of your child and her self-injury, you can also look for indirect evidence that first-aid supplies are being used (e.g., you can track the number of adhesive bandages, gauze, or cotton swabs that are used in any given time period. You can also check your child's trash for evidence of used first-aid supplies). However, if you suspect that your child is still self-injuring, we encourage you to refrain from using what you know (or suspect) to confront her about it. Gathering this information is more of an opportunity for you to pay attention to trends over time. Throwing it at her during a confrontation or argument is only going to lead to feelings of betrayal and resentment in your child, driving a wedge between the two of you. Hopefully, you'll see a reduction in signs of self-injury shortly. Once parents and their children become more comfortable being honest with each other, parents may be more likely to receive more accurate and honest responses from their children when they ask.

> If you suspect that your child is still self-injuring, we encourage you to refrain from using what you know (or suspect) to confront her about it.

One additional note of caution here: for most people, self-injury is about control and regaining control of their emotions. Parents may also find themselves wanting to take control of the situation by instilling strict rules and policies in the house, such as requiring children to show their arms or other body parts for signs of fresh injuries. If you aim to take away all privacy or access to normal household items (scissors, knives, etc.), this may work against you and leave your child feeling more out of control and helpless (Chapter 12 discusses more fully safety concerns and no-harm contracts). Once parents and their children become more comfortable being very honest with each other, you may feel more inclined to ask for—and more likely to receive—more accurate and honest responses from your child.

Significant and Consistent Changes in Mood

As you know by now, self-injury is often used as a way to shift moods and gain control over feelings. People who self-injure may appear moody or may display many more negative than positive mood states. In this case, reduced volatility of moods is a clear indicator of important and positive change. It is important to note that there are a number of people who self-injure who do not present outwardly as depressed, anxious, or emotionally withdrawn. Some people are masterful at masking negative moods through hyper-engagement in activity and/or constantly upbeat or "can-do" orientations. They may actually be using self-injury as a way to keep their moods stable. In these cases, individuals may present as always on, connected, or engaged, and improvements would be evidenced through more natural, moderate, "up-and-down" mood states that are neither overly dramatic or exaggerated. One subtle but sure sign of change is when your child responds more positively or authentically in a stressful situation than he or she might otherwise have responded. This can be one of the earliest signs of productive change.

Increases in Optimistic or Positive Comments or Expectations

People who self-injure often report many more negative than positive thoughts. These can be critical of self or others. They can also reflect negative expectations about performance, other people's perceptions, or life possibilities. While the content of these negative comments is important, what's also important is the *balance* of negative to positive statements and the overall valence, or potency, of the associated emotions. Marked shifts in the ratio of these indicate significant change, as do comments with less emotional charge than normal. Beyond this, noticing the areas of life in which positivity is creeping in is also important and a telling sign that a person is feeling safer emotionally. Increased positivity and change in the expectations for one's life and one's self-esteem are the areas likely to drive the greatest behavioral shifts.

Changes in Activity Levels and Focus

If self-injury behaviors become persistent and common, engagement in other healthy life activities may decrease. This is not necessarily a result of the self-injury, per se, but of the inner emotional or cognitive discomfort self-injury signals. You will know that he or she is starting to heal and will see a shift in willingness to engage in other healthy

> Watch for greater engagement in positive and helpful activities—it's a clear sign of progress even if the self-injury has not stopped altogether or even slowed down much.

life activities. Watch for greater engagement in positive and helpful activities—it's a clear sign of progress even if the self-injury has not stopped altogether or even slowed down much. As with other changes, people usually begin experimenting with new ways of thinking, feeling, and doing in areas of life that feel the least risky.

Improvement in Relationships

When someone is self-injuring, it is common to pull away from relationships outside, particularly with people who might be able to clue in to the inner turmoil and ask about it. Close family members—those on the front line—are often the first people to feel this detachment. Close friends, other relatives, or important adults may also be on the receiving end of this detachment. Improvements in any of these close relationships, such as spending more time together, having more honest conversations, or engaging in shared activities are clear signs of improvement and healing.

What Is Not Helpful

> *Don't tell them that what they are doing is wrong. They know what they are doing is wrong.*
> —Rachel, reflecting on her past serious self-injury

What is *not* helpful is focusing on failures or continued negative patterns related to self-injury. While parents cannot ignore these, and while there do need to be consequences for violations of agreements, we strongly recommend doing this quietly and with as little strong emotion as possible. We devoted Section 4 of the book to communicating effectively with your child, building an empathic and supportive relationship, and setting clear and effective boundaries. Save your strong emotions for expressions of positive emotion—love, support, encouragement, confidence, and validation. The magnitude of emotion is as powerful as the emotion itself. While it may not be possible to stop yourself from having a negative, discouraged reaction to something, aim to keep from reacting loudly or repeatedly referring back to it.

Preventing Burnout

Knowing that there will be light at the end of the tunnel only goes so far in helping parents remain calm and compassionate for themselves, their children, and other family members along the way. Indeed, there is often a strong tendency for parents to be so focused on assuring their children's well-being that they do not seek adequate support for themselves. Virtually all parents report feeling unhappy, worrying about their child's future, feeling emotionally strained and tired, and feeling like their child's self-injury has taken a significant toll on their family.[6]

Every parent with whom we have spoken about their child's self-injury clearly communicates his or her care and concern. And yet, while the child may be in therapy, many parents had not considered therapy for themselves, nor had they told others about their challenges. This prevents them from gaining valuable emotional support. Self-injury not only creates fertile ground for high levels of stress, but it can also lead to guilt, self-judgment, feelings of confusion, and social isolation. Moreover, the "on and off again" nature of the behavior can add a dimension of uncertainty that heightens feelings of emotional and existential insecurity about the future well-being of your child and family.

When we measure secondary stress in caregivers, we typically focus on three different types. The first is the logistical stress and strain that can come with having to deal with the various accommodations (e.g., transportation and costs of therapy appointments, disrupted family routines) that have to be made, as well as the impact on time, money, and other tangible resources. The second kind of strain is emotional in nature and relates to the feelings of resentment, anger, or fear about your child and concerns about his or her future. The third kind of strain is also emotional in nature and relates to the negative emotions you may have that are directed at yourself, through feelings of worry, guilt, or anger. Research has shown that parents of children who self-injure are more likely to feel uncertain about how to parent effectively, especially with regard to managing conflict and communication problems. They are also likely to worry that their parenting approaches will trigger more or worse self-injury episodes. All of these are common and understandable.

You might provide logistical and financial support for your child to receive therapy and possible in-patient services. You'll also provide crucial emotional support to your child, who is clearly struggling with strong emotions and life changes. But, as parents, you are not just supporters, allies, and logistics coordinators. Even more important than the logistics role you play in keeping your eye on the big picture is the longer term vision—that is, modeling how to express and manage strong emotions and thoughts and staying as balanced and healthy as you can through it all. Learning how to do all of these things, especially soon after finding out about the depth of your child's suffering, is a journey all its own. It helps to be patient with yourself and to stay aware that there is always time to adjust course as needed. As one parent shared:

> At first it caused us to hover, shelter, and stifle because we were so scared. We were completely caught off guard. We overcompensated, lowered expectations, and babied . . . most of these things were more detrimental than helpful. In some ways, I feel we were too entangled. I thought I needed to be her support all the time, it was exhausting and a crutch to her. With lots of reading and a good family therapist, we learned and are still learning to set appropriate boundaries and to let her learn . . . to stop rescuing her. If she cuts, we didn't cause it, she is learning to deal with her feelings. . . . Boundaries and rules are vital and part of parenting. If you are parenting out of fear and always lowering the bar, you aren't helping your child. We are all learning and growing.
>
> —*Tamir, parent of an adolescent who self-injures*

There is evidence that the emotional states of those you care for or with whom you spend a lot of time can actually be somewhat contagious (called "social contagion" or "emotional mimicry"). For this reason, it is particularly vital that you engage in a lot of self-care. As we all know, it's very hard to help someone when you're also experiencing distress. One of the most common reflections we hear from families is how instrumental professional support was to their personal well-being in a stressful time. Thus, seeking support and advice early is critical.

Professionals also advise seeking support early. At first, this support is likely to focus on getting information about self-injury and associated problems and about how to connect one's child to professional support. After this, however, support for parents is immensely helpful in navigating the bumpy process of change. Since emotions and situations may become worse before they start to improve, parents are strongly encouraged to line up a support system, formal and/or informal, to turn to when life is confusing or difficult. We talk a great deal about this in Chapter 13.

> I sent myself a lifeline. I have learned to manage my depression and anxiety through treatment and therapy. My life is no longer ruled by my emotions, and my ability to function in relationships and work has improved as I mature. Treatments have improved a great deal, and I am hopeful that better options will exist for my daughters, both of whom struggle, that will give them a better quality of life.
>
> —Lita, mother of two daughters who self-injure and who also has a self-injury history

> Finding a good therapeutic team that we trusted was really important. Family therapy has really been important, mostly for us to not fear being a parent. Because initially you have guilt and you think you somehow caused this and you are afraid you will cause your child to harm himself if you set boundaries. I think it is vital that you release guilt or you can end up providing secondary benefits that reinforce the behavior you are trying to help overcome. Lastly, you learn to provide love and support, but also respect the knowledge that you can't fix it for them. I know we will all get through this, just not as quickly as we want.
>
> —Avila, mother of a son who self-injures

Taking the Long View

> Seems like we take two steps forward and then many steps back.
> The self-harm is an addictive behavior now, and I am realizing that

I cannot fix it. Only she can, and I am not sure she wants to fix anything.

—Ben, father of a daughter who self-injures

We wish we could tell you that once you read this book and put local supports in place, things will resolve quickly. That may happen, but it may not. Change can take time and growth and struggle. As parents and professionals, it has helped us to *take the long view*. It may be helpful to keep in mind that the mere experience of growing up and getting older will iron out some of the wrinkles with which you and your child struggle. The more challenges that are present, the longer this can take, but even people with serious mental illness can and do learn how to cope reasonably well over time. Section 4 of this book offers lots of practical suggestions and examples of how to help your child navigate the process of changing self-injury behavior while strengthening your relationship with one another. For now, please consider the following important suggestions that can be useful for framing your thinking about self-injury and how to take the long view.

Tips for How To Take the Long View

- *Stopping self-injury doesn't happen until the person who needs to stop is ready.* The most essential ingredients of healing are wanting to stop and being ready to find other ways of coping. This is often the most difficult issue for parents because, although they can provide a lot of support, they cannot provide the desire to stop nor the will to change. You may be very ready for things to change, but that will not matter unless your child is also authentically ready.
- *The urge to self-injure can be very powerful.* At first, those trying to change their self-injury behavior are likely to find that other methods of coping don't work as well or as fast as self-injury does. The urge to self-injure can be very strong. When someone learns to notice these desires early and actively chooses to engage other patterns of coping instead, he or she creates new neurological patterns, a process that strengthens the capacity to reduce reliance on self-injury and increases the

ability to employ more healthy ways of managing stress and other triggers.

- *Slips and relapses are common.* Knowing this ahead of time can be helpful in staying focused on the big picture. Rather than seeing a slip as failure, view it as a learning opportunity. It's a chance to reflect on why the slip happened and to try to understand what led your child to be vulnerable in this situation. This can help reduce risk of the same thing happening in the future. It requires becoming a scholar of oneself—an individual wanting to stop injuring will need to collect subtle and often detailed "data" about what feelings, thoughts, and contexts trigger his self-injury, and, if he is doing deeper work, how he arrived at a place in life where self-injury became an option. You'll find lots of content in this book that aims to help you uncover your child's "triggers" for self-injury and how these may relate to your own thoughts and feelings. For instance, Chapters 7 and 9 discuss how you can use an Automatic Thoughts Record to help uncover connections between your thoughts, feelings, and behaviors. Chapters 9 and 10 help you to use this newfound information about yourself and your child to develop mindful parenting skills, thus strengthening your ability to communicate and connect in a meaningful way.

- *The "dry drunk" phenomenon: this happens in self-injury, too.* In the Alcoholics Anonymous community, a "dry drunk" is someone who has stopped drinking but who still relies on many of the same thought and feeling patterns. This most often comes out as negativity, pessimism, anger, and avoidance. Individuals who leave the behavior behind but don't change their internal landscape are at high risk of relapsing or replacing the drinking with other harmful behaviors. The same thing can happen in self-injury. The goal is, of course, to help your child to not need to self-injure, but ultimately this means taking a hard look at what's behind the self-injury (i.e., the thoughts and feelings that might be contributing to the need to self-injure) and to find safer and healthier ways to manage these.

- *Time is on your side.* Since the relationships among emotions, thoughts, and behaviors naturally undergo significant change in adolescence and early adulthood, time and natural development are often allies. Young adults' ability to regulate mood and emotions is going to be markedly better than it was when they were in their young or middle adolescence, regardless of what else is going on. The difficulty is in the fact that neurological patterns can become quite habitual. As evidenced by the phrase in the scientific community "neurons that fire together, wire together," our brains are easily trained to link specific thoughts, emotions, and behavioral reactions together (for example, "I think that I am a failure—I feel sad and distressed—I self-injure"). Once these are in place, establishing other, healthier thought patterns requires time and effort, a task which tends to become easier with age (see Chapter 10 for more on how to do this).

Activities

Activity 1: The Nuts and Bolts of Healing: A Checklist for Noticing Improvement

We encourage you to complete this checklist on a weekly basis or as often as you see fit. If your child is in the early stages of change (Moratorium, Awareness, Preparation), it may be better for you to complete this on your own. Once your child has moved into more active healing and is engaged in rebuilding, it may be helpful to review this checklist with him or her and see if he or she has interest in using it. Regardless of their children's interest, parents will benefit from completing this checklist as a way to gauge progress toward healthy change. We hope the checklist will be helpful for noting your observations about small changes you are observing.

	Improvement	No change	Decline	Notes
Self-injury behavior				
Number of incidents				
Severity of self-injury				
Other:				
Emotion & mood				
Constructively expressed emotion				

	Improvement	No change	Decline	Notes
Showed positive emotion/mood				
Positive reaction to good news, events, social exchange or opportunities				
Clear use of new ways of coping with emotion				
Thoughts				
Clearly expressed positive thoughts about self				
Clearly expressed positive thoughts about others				
Clearly stated thoughts about goals/future				

	Improvement	No change	Decline	Notes
Engagement in activities				
Participated in healthy activities				
Showed interest or engaged in new healthy activities				
Social relationships				
Showed interest in healthy relationships with friends				
Showed interest in healthy relationships with family members				
Showed interest in healthy relationships with other relationships (teachers, etc.)				
Invested in new healthy relationships				

Activity 2: Reflection Activity

Consider what you have learned about the stages of self-injury change and respond to the following:

1. What stage of change do you feel that your child is in?

   _____

   _____

   _____

   _____

   _____

2. Identify two concrete steps that you can take to better communicate with and/or help your child in his or her healing efforts:

   _____

   _____

   _____

   _____

   _____

3. Identify two concrete steps that your child may be able to take right now to help him- or herself:

   _____

   _____

   _____

   _____

   _____

An Introduction to Therapy

Talking with Your Child About Therapy and Finding the Right Therapist

[T]he key to anyone going to therapy? You have to want to go. You can't force someone to go to AA, you can't force someone to want to feel better. They have to want to feel better.

—Ben, father of a youth who self-injures

What Do We Know About the Course of Self-Injury During Adolescence?

For some teens, self-injury can be simply an "experiment," occurring just a few times and then never again (perhaps even unknown to their families). For many others, their experimentation can be the beginning of a long road that can stretch for years, perhaps happening sporadically, with weeks, months, or even years between episodes. This is not so dissimilar to teens' relationships with drugs, with some experimenting a few times and never again, while others keep going back and dramatically alter the course of their lives.

Unfortunately, despite our best research efforts, there are no clear and predictable pathways to anticipating who will experiment with self-injury—or any other addictive habit, like substance abuse—and who will go on to regularly use these strategies to cope. Even once someone starts injuring, it is impossible to predict who will experiment once or twice and then discontinue on his own and who will likely engage in it repetitively and end up needing therapeutic support to stop.

The good news is that the brain development taking place during adolescence and young adulthood allows for cognitive growth and social maturity. These changes, what we all call "growing up," can foster not only new skills, but insight into why the self-injuring began in the first place, the various functions it serves, and what the individual needs to stop the behavior for good. Indeed, in one of our studies, nearly one-third of those who were no longer self-injuring described new self-awareness, coping skills, and other healthy changes in their life circumstances.[1]

Does Seeking Help Really Help? Changing the Course of Nonsuicidal Self-Injury

While not every individual who engages in nonsuicidal self-injury (NSSI) also has other mental health challenges, a large majority of them do. Most commonly, self-injury can occur alongside symptoms of depression, anxiety, stress, anger, difficulties with regulating emotions, borderline personality symptoms, and suicidal thoughts and behaviors.[2] Professional support is helpful in navigating all of the things that tend to come up as your child works to change self-injury behavior.

Critical Elements of Effective Psychological Therapy

As you begin to learn more about the various forms of psychological therapy available, it is easy to become overwhelmed by the details of what each therapy aims to accomplish. However, there are common elements across all effective psychological therapies that are key to their success. Regardless of the name or the type of therapy or the letters after the therapist's name, these elements are important to successfully identifying and managing self-injury thoughts and behaviors. We call these out here because these are also approaches you can use at home, in less structured ways, of course. We will come back to how to use these in the last section of this book.

Key Elements of Therapy

- *Ongoing assessment of risk factors and triggers*: A thorough assessment involves an initial evaluation by the clinician focused on self-injury behaviors (what, when, where, with whom), along with the emotions and physiological responses that lead up to ("triggers") and follow self-injury behaviors.[3] A therapist may ask that the client record her thoughts, feelings, and self-injury behaviors throughout therapy. The goal is to educate both the therapist *and* client on the factors and triggers that lead to self-injury or the desire to self-injure. Bringing awareness to these triggers allows for more opportunity to step in and break the cycle of self-harm.
- *Skills training*: All psychotherapy techniques involve *skills training*, most often addressing thoughts and behaviors that contribute to and help to maintain the self-injury. For instance, all modalities include strategies for how to begin addressing negative thoughts (called "self-talk") and how to best manage unhelpful behavior patterns that are part of self-harm patterns. Many therapies also commonly include problem-solving as a strategy. Some emphasize this element more than others, but being able to identify problem situations ahead of time, generate possible solutions, and implement solutions effectively are important skills from which many who engage in self-injury can benefit.
- *Targeting and strengthening relationships:* Youth who self-injure commonly report and demonstrate troubles in key relationships and in their responses to interpersonal difficulties.[4] If you are reading this book, you clearly have an interest in doing what you can to help your child—and yourself—grow and become stronger from these experiences. Improving and strengthening relationships may take many forms depending on what is needed for a particular individual and may include social skills training, effective communication

strategies, interpreting social cues, and learning which relationships are healthy and which are unhealthy when it comes to stopping self-injuring.

- *Identifying and addressing other unhealthy, maladaptive behaviors*: While not all teens who engage in self-injury also experience other psychological difficulties, a high proportion of self-injuring teens do. The most common of these are substance abuse (e.g., alcohol, nicotine, marijuana), eating disorders, depression and anxiety (e.g., posttraumatic stress disorder, generalized anxiety), and conduct or oppositional disorders. Indeed, one study found that 87% of a sample of *hospitalized* teens engaging in self-injury met criteria for a mental illness diagnosis.[5] Thus, it becomes important to address these other behaviors, how they may relate to self-injury, and what underlying factors are common (such as difficulty tolerating strong emotions or distress and feeling emotionally out of control). These factors then become targets for treatment.

Regardless of the lack of consensus about what treatment approaches are most effective in what circumstances, one thing remains clear: *relationships truly matter to the process of healing.* Treatment of self-injury involves working on building healthy, supportive relationships with others while also addressing unhealthy ways of coping and managing uncomfortable emotions.

> Relationships truly matter to the process of healing.

Talking with Your Child About Therapy

It is common for parents to find themselves anxious and stressed about the prospect of seeking formal therapy. The idea of sharing very personal thoughts and experiences, some of which may be associated with painful family memories, can bring up feelings of shame or fear. Stigma around seeking therapy can run very deep. Moreover, if anyone in the household has attended therapy but found it less than useful, there may be added disincentive to seek formal support now.

Nevertheless, most people who use NSSI regularly to cope with stress will need formal therapeutic support. And most people who successfully change chronic self-injury report therapy as an important part of the healing process.[6] In addition to parental support, a strong therapeutic alliance (e.g., good relationships with a therapist) is instrumental in successful treatment. For this reason, in families with more than one parent, it is often helpful for parents to discuss their perspectives on therapy with one another. The goal is to arrive at some degree of consensus about how to speak in a unified manner about what parents see as the need for and expectations of therapy.

Discussing expectations with a child about attending therapy can be challenging. Self-injury is often tough to treat, and it is not uncommon for people who self-injure to dislike therapy or a particular therapist because they feel too pushed or not well understood. This is particularly true in the earlier stages of change, when the idea of stopping a behavior that helps one feel better is very threatening. Ironically, being challenged in this way often ends up being one of the aspects of therapy that individuals who self-injure later cite as *helpful*. But the timing and exact nature of such challenges are critically linked to readiness to change, and this is why having a therapist who is able to form a good "therapeutic alliance" with your child (and/or other members of the family) is so helpful. This, however, can take time to establish. As a result, resistance to therapy is often a normal but stressful experience for families. Not wanting to start therapy, missing appointments, or refusing to go anymore are all common. This can be especially disconcerting for parents because they may think of therapy as a beacon of hope, maybe the *only* beacon of hope.

To begin a conversation with your child about therapy, consider the following tips:

- *Be clear about your expectations:* Be very clear about what you expect to get out of therapy and share these expectations with your child. Acknowledge that you recognize that his goals and your goals may be different. A good therapist will work in close alignment with your child's goals while keeping the parental goals in mind as well.
- *Avoid blaming your child for the self-injury; help her understand that the therapy is to support her goals, not*

yours: Assure your child that you are not blaming her, punishing her, or sending her to therapy in order to stop self-injuring (otherwise she is likely to feel like she is going to therapy for you, not for herself, and this does not work). Tell her that the goal is give her an outside support person to talk to, someone who is not so close to the things in her life that are causing stress. Tell her that you believe that professional support can help her figure out what she wants for her life and how to get it in healthy ways.

- *Encourage your child to take an active role in the process*: Assure your child that he is not going to be stuck with someone he does not like; that he can "interview" therapists to find the best fit. In small communities with few eligible therapists, this may be less possible, but where there is more than one possible therapist, it is a great idea to meet with more than one so that your child feels like he has choices.

- *Try to avoid thinking of therapy as a "cure"*: Know that seeing a therapist is not necessarily the cure-all that parents may desire. As we've discussed, stopping self-injury can be messy and can take time, with stops and starts along the way. Parents will need to carefully and honestly reflect on why they want their child to seek therapy, paying particular attention to any beliefs that a therapist will be able to "fix" a child in a 1-hour, once-a-week session, and all a parent needs to do is drive him or her to the appointments.

There will be instances in which a child is so deeply resistant to therapy that you question whether it would be useful. In some cases, the resistance will be so constant that therapy probably won't be useful. That said, it may be important to have engaging in therapy as one of your bottom-line requirements for your child. A good therapist can work with even resistant people by not pushing them too hard to make changes they are not ready to make. Moreover, there are many interesting techniques in practice now, using art, music, meditation, and other forms of self-expression as a way to creatively express what cannot be spoken so well. Whether or not to force therapy is a decision you and your family will have to make, but in instances where you decide or know it is necessary, do whatever you can to allow your child to have as much involvement in the process and the choice of therapist as possible.

Taking an Active Role in Treatment: Finding the Right Therapist

Finding the right therapist is important. In some cases, therapy can be unhelpful or can even make things worse. In cases where the patient–therapist fit is poor, where the therapy techniques are not well-suited to the patient's readiness to change, or where the youth uses the sessions to reinforce his or her narrative about why self-injury is necessary can lead to nonproductive therapy at best and detrimental therapy at worst. One parent describes a series of missteps in the care her daughter received from various mental health professionals:

> The worst experience we had was how her middle and high school therapists and school social workers handled the situation. The judgment of others was cruel and inefficient. Her father continues to be in denial although he is a social worker as well. She had the strength and support to fire her therapists as needed and has found the talk therapy that supports her goals and aims. She just got off antidepressant meds after a year of exploring psychiatric intervention, she has discovered that she is her best resource in combination with talking to others openly and honestly—namely me, her sister, and brother.
>
> —*Jen, parent of young woman who self-injures*

In one of our studies, more than half of teens and young adults who self-injure described experiences in which they worked with a therapist they did not find helpful.[7] This can be explained in a few ways. First, these instances could certainly be related to a poor "fit" with a therapist. It is possible that the therapist may not have been comfortable or trained properly to work with an individual who is self-injuring. It is important that communities have therapists who are comfortable dealing with this issue, as well as "get to know you" sessions where clients and therapists are able to assess whether the fit is good. Second, some young people consider therapy to be unhelpful when struggling with whether they really wants to quit injuring. Therapy requires a lot or emotional work at times, and it may be easier for your child to say that

Individuals are much more likely to see therapy as helpful in retrospect, after they are well into or have completed the therapeutic process.

the therapist wasn't helpful rather than admit that he didn't want to change his behavior and the thoughts and emotions conneted to it. Indeed, our studies in this area show that individuals are much more likely to see therapy as helpful in retrospect, after they are well into or have completed the therapeutic process, than they are to view therapy as helpful while actively engaged in self-injury.

Obstacles to Seeking Treatment

Once the decision to seek therapy has been made, it is important to know that you may meet a few obstacles along the path of identifying the treatment most likely to meet your needs. One of the most common barriers is gathering enough strength to mobilize the emotional resources and knowledge needed to locate a treatment provider. As one parent noted, "I am so overwhelmed that I don't know how to find the help I need so badly."

It's not uncommon for parents to report not knowing what to do or what steps to take first. Reaching out to your child's pediatrician or primary care provider may offer leads for local therapists, as will contacting your health insurance provider to see if they can provide you with a list of mental health clinicians in your area who work with adolescents. The American Psychological Association also offers a resource for locating therapists in your area: apa.org/helpcenter/choose-therapist.aspx.

> It's not uncommon for parents to report not knowing what to do or what steps to take first.

For those with limited access to local therapists or therapists skilled in the types of therapies most helpful for self-injury (see the next chapter for details), new resources for counseling are becoming available on the Internet, such as talkspace.com, which does not offer counseling services for people below the age of 18 but can be really helpful for parents who want flexibility in when and how they participate in therapy for themselves. Other web- and phone-based applications are increasingly common as well. The apps Talk Life and 7 Cups of Tea, for example, offers a variety of supports, including formal online therapy. Both of these are highly utilized by youth. In these cases, however, engagement of the family is less common, and so parents may feel much less aware of a child's progress.

There are also practical issues relating to having the necessary time and money for treatment. While most contemporary insurance packages cover mental health treatment, not all do. Providers have various treatment programs, so it is always good to check out the possibilities. Also, community-based providers, such as children and family services or offices of mental health services run by the state or county, can offer therapy at a reduced rate in situations where there is financial hardship.

It's also important that know what you are committing to with a particular form of therapy or services. We encourage you to use the Finding the Right Therapist Checklist as a guide to finding a therapist who is right for your child and/or family, your values, and your resources. It is critical that you ask questions—and get answers—that help you to determine whether a particular treatment may meet your child's and your family's needs.

Activities

A Checklist for Finding the Right Therapist for You and Your Child

In light of the many options available, finding a therapist to help with managing various life experiences and challenges has never been easier. Nevertheless, finding the right one for you, one who has experience working with youth who self-injure and their families, may be more challenging. Here are a few things to consider when you decide that the time is right to seek some professional guidance and support.

- ☐ Do you (and your teen) feel safe and comfortable talking with the therapist? Is the person down-to-earth or does he or she feel cold and emotionally removed? Only you can decide whether there is a good fit or not. There is no rule that requires you to continue working with a counselor. However, Noah Rubinstein, founder of goodtherapy.org, recommends that you be honest with yourself and your feelings: "It's important to check to see if there's a part of you avoiding therapy through a dislike or judgment of the therapist. If you find yourself reacting negatively to every counselor you see, then the issue could be yours and may warrant your sticking it out with a counselor in an effort to work through your fears of beginning therapy."

- ☐ What's the therapist's general philosophy and approach to helping? Does your therapist approach people in a compassionate and optimistic way? Is she open-minded? Issues related to how she views life—and whether that is consistent with your own views and values—are important to consider as you look for a therapist that will fit your needs. It's easy to go with the therapist who has the best online reviews, but it's more important to go with what's best for you personally.

- ☐ Does the therapist have experience helping youth who self-injure? Has he helped other families with a loved one who is self-injuring? The more experience a therapist has addressing a particular issue, concern, or problem area, the more expertise he has developed.

- Does the therapist offer you a (relatively) clear plan on how she intends to set about helping you and/or your child? Experienced therapists should be able to provide you with information on how they believe treatment should be structured, how often it should occur, and what they would be looking for as measures of "success."

- Is the therapist licensed? Licensure generally implies that therapists have received many hours of training and education in their field (whether it be counseling, psychology or psychiatry, social work, or marriage and family therapy). They will have completed the required hours of training in order to sit for their licensing exam and will be required by the state to complete a certain number of continuing education credits each year in order to stay up to date in their field.

Therapy for Self-Injury

What helped? Finding a good therapeutic team that we trust, knowing we are providing her with as many tools as we can, and trusting she will figure this out and accepting that we may not be perfect, that we didn't cause this and that we have to accept where we all are in the process. Family therapy has been important, mostly for us to not fear being a parent. Because initially you have guilt and you think you somehow caused this and you are afraid you will cause your child to take away their stressors without enabling them.

—Niska, mother to a daughter who self-injures

I think our relationship is stronger now partly I believe because I did not give up on her. We continued to seek therapy until we found something that worked (this has taken over 2 years)

—Anu, father of a daughter who self-injures

Considering a Stepped-Care Approach to Therapy

Should a teen who has experimented with self-injury a few times receive the same amount and type of therapy as someone who has engaged in self-injury for a year or more? A stepped-care approach to treating self-injury argues against a "one-size-fits-all" strategy, instead matching patient needs with the most appropriate type and amount of therapy.[1]

Stepped-care is an important organizational system aimed at benefiting teens and their families. It also helps therapists to determine what services may be most appropriate for the situation. Depending on the length of time a teen has engaged in self-injury, the severity and frequency of self-harm behaviors, other unhealthy behaviors that may be occurring (such as substance abuse), and the degree of family support available to the teen, levels of therapeutic care will be more or less intensive in nature. They may involve weekly sessions with an outpatient therapist or could be utilized in inpatient facilities and involve multiple family and individual sessions each week.

Any clinician you work with should be open to discussing with you issues related to a stepped-care approach to helping your teen. Important questions to discuss with your potential therapist as you consider your child's (and family's) needs include:

- How much treatment do you and your child want?
- How often are you willing to commit to therapy appointments?
- How much are you willing or able to pay?
- How much work are you willing to put in during and between treatment sessions?

In combination with your teen's experience of self-injury, your answers to these questions will help guide you and the therapist in determining an overall treatment plan for your child that realistically takes into account the frequency and length of services and in what way your family should be integrated into therapy. What services are available in the area and your family's financial situation should also be considered.

Clients usually move through less intensive interventions before receiving more intensive interventions if they are necessary. As the intensity of the self-injury behavior increases, so, too, would the level of care. Various levels of therapy intensity range from education/prevention efforts in school settings, to brief individual therapy, longer term individual and family therapy, and the use of medications and intensive residential treatment. Stepped levels of care and who may be appropriate for each are briefly outlined here:

- *Step 1*: Youth who have just begun hurting themselves may benefit from a Step 1 approach. This would consist of a detailed assessment by a trained professional to evaluate the factors that might contribute to self-harm behaviors as well as to establish a behavioral contract that sets goals for reducing/ eliminating nonsuicidal self-injury (NSSI) by replacing self-harm behaviors with other more adaptive skills and rewarding themselves for reaching their goals.
- *Step 2*: Teens experiencing recurring self-injury of low lethality may benefit from all Step 1 components *plus* the addition of cognitive-behavioral therapy, family therapy, and, if needed, psychopharmacological treatment.
- *Step 3*: Teens engaging in persistent self-injury and also suffering from suicidal thoughts, posttraumatic stress disorder, an eating disorder, or substance abuse may need a more intensive Step 3 level of care. This would involve all previously described components plus the addition of care for these other mental health issues and possibly hospitalization for safety.
- *Step 4*: Teens with serious mental illness, especially psychosis, and who may be involved in multiple self-destructive behaviors may benefit from a highly structured approach called *illness management and recovery* (IMR). This structured recovery model emphasizes personal choice and focuses on recovery strategies, identifying symptoms and warning signs, using the stress-vulnerability model, building social support, using medications effectively, reducing relapse, improved coping with stress, and the role that drugs and/or alcohol may play in the experience of symptoms.

This chapter aims to provide you with information on the most effective psychological treatments available for managing self-injury. Regardless of the level of care your child may receive, she will likely be engaged in one or more of these forms of therapy.

Psychological Therapy for Self-Injury

There are four primary forms of psychotherapy for self-injury that have scientific evidence to support them: *family-based therapy, cognitive-behavioral therapy, problem-solving therapy,* and *dialectical behavior therapy.* These are described next, along with the scientific evidence that supports their effectiveness. It is important to note that all of these treatments can be used in both outpatient mental health settings as well as inpatient hospital and residential settings, although hospital, residential, and day program settings often involve more frequent (and perhaps intensive) therapy. Most of the research exploring the effectiveness of various treatments is based on studies of clients receiving outpatient therapy. Unfortunately, very few studies exist looking at the effectiveness of hospital and residential therapy for self-injury.

It's also important to note that not all of these therapies were designed initially for the specific treatment of self-injury. Over the years, they have been modified to meet the needs of clients who self-injure. While these treatments are commonly used in mental health settings, there is still a need for systematic research studies, the most trusted of which are randomized controlled trials (RCT).

> Unfortunately, very few studies have evaluated the effectiveness of treatments for self-injuring youth.

When it comes to scientific measurement of whether a drug or a therapy technique is effective at helping people, the RCT is the gold standard. An RCT assigns participants to receive one of two or more forms of treatment (in the case of medication trials, often without them knowing which they're receiving) and compares those participants receiving treatment A with those receiving treatment B, C, and so on, typically following them for months and sometimes years to see what works. You have probably heard of RCTs for medical drug trials where one group of people receives the medical drug being tested and another group does not, but no one in either group knows whether they are receiving the actual medication or the *placebo* (either no treatment or a recognized medication that the new drug is being compared to). Similar kinds of studies can be conducted to test whether therapy techniques are helpful in treating challenges like self-injury. Where information on RCTs for self-injury is available, we provide it. Unfortunately, *very few* studies have evaluated the effectiveness of treatments for self-injuring youth. So, where appropriate, we will also mention RCTs that include adults or those that have engaged in self-harm with *suicidal* intent. Another confounding factor when examining RCTs is their use of a comparison condition often labeled "treatment as usual." This is meant to reflect the type of services that an individual might receive if she were to seek out mental health care from a professional in her community (such as providing referrals as needed or monitoring for signs of distress). Obviously, this can vary widely, and so it's difficult to know what services study participants are actually receiving if they are assigned to "treatment as usual" in a RCT.

We admit that the research on treatments for NSSI is confounding and frustrating because so little exists from which we can draw solid conclusions. This is an area in which science and its research-intensive methods must catch up with the needs of the community. Until then, we must draw conclusions from the information that we have available (Table 7.1).

Family-Based Therapy

What is it and how does it work? Family-focused or family-based therapy (FBT) is founded on the idea that individual functioning reflects, in part, the larger health (or lack of health) of a family system.[2] Even when individual mental health difficulties cannot be clearly traced to family dynamics, there is abundant evidence to suggest that how families relate to and manage this crisis can make a big difference in the child's healing process. For this reason, family-based therapy targets improvements in family functioning and cohesiveness through education on psychological processes, communication training, and problem-solving. With respect to self-injury, family

Table 7.1 Critical Elements of Common Nonsuicidal Self-Injury Psychological Therapies

	Assesses risk factors and triggers	Promotes skills training	Targets and strengthens relationships	Identifies and addresses other unhealthy behaviors
Cognitive-Behavioral Therapy (CBT)	X	X	½	X
Dialectical Behavior Therapy (DBT)	X	X	X	X
Problem-Solving Therapy (PST)	X	X	½	½
Family-Based Therapy (FBT)	X	X	X	½

½= possesses some of this quality but not all of it

therapy is intended to educate families about the purpose(s) that self-injury serves for the teen, decrease behaviors within the family that may trigger self-injury, define the roles that parents and teens play within the family, and decrease emotional outbursts and improve communication around family members' internal emotional landscapes.

Why should families be targeted so directly in the treatment of a teen's self-injury? There is extensive research indicating that family factors such as poor family communication, excessive parental criticism, loss of a caregiver, and mental health issues in first-degree relatives are risk factors for all forms of teen self-harm.[3] Adolescents often say that family conflict triggers self-injury. Indeed, some research indicates that parent relationships play a more powerful role than peer relationships when it comes to thoughts of suicide, even during the teenage years.[4] Multiple studies have emphasized the powerful role of parents in ending self-injury and in reducing the likelihood of considering or attempting suicide.[5] Parents and other family members can know-

> Multiple studies have emphasized the powerful role of parents in ending self-injury and in reducing likelihood of considering or attempting suicide.

ingly, or unknowingly, worsen self-injury behavior by expressing critical or hostile remarks, becoming emotionally overinvolved, or consciously choosing to distance themselves from their teens. This can set the stage for teens to avoid seeking support when they need it most.

Does it work? One study evaluated the effectiveness of FBT by aiming to reduce suicidal thoughts and behaviors by improving the parent–teen relationship.[6] Families were randomly assigned to receive either cognitive-behavioral family sessions held weekly over 3 months or treatment as usual. While NSSI was not specifically evaluated, results indicated that teens receiving FBT reported much less suicidal ideation over the course of the 3 months of treatment, with depression symptoms also declining. Would self-injury and suicidal behaviors also decrease with this treatment? Unfortunately, the study didn't measure these, although the results are promising.

Another study of FBT focused specifically on parent training only.[7] The goal was to increase families' knowledge about self-harm thoughts and behaviors, improve parenting practices, and decrease family conflict and stress. Indeed, adolescents from families receiving this brief (four-session) parent training intervention reported fewer self-injury and suicide-related thoughts and behaviors. These results are promising and suggest the need for additional research examining FBT and parent-training studies.

Not all individuals who self-injure will want or need family treatment. Some may want to focus exclusively on individual therapy, while others may not have family members who want to be involved in therapy. For others, family treatment may not be immediately warranted, with individual treatment to better manage and express emotions being necessary before family sessions can be productive. In short, FBTs are not a one-size-fits-all approach and can vary in emphasis and techniques, with some focusing on attachment issues between parents and teens, some focusing solely on parents, and some taking a narrower, very problem-focused approach that targets self-injury only. In general, the question of whether or not family therapy will be helpful is best answered by the therapists who are connected to the family. Once the therapist has a sense of how family dynamics may be contributing to the problem and or how they can contribute to the solution, she is likely to reach out and suggest this. Additionally, you as the parent can initiate the process with the therapist by asking her impression of its usefulness.

Cognitive-Behavioral Therapy

What is it and how does it work? Cognitive behavioral therapy (CBT) is the most widely used evidence-based psychological intervention for improving a wide range of mental health issues. Developed in the 1960s, CBT targets the relationship that an individual has with his or her negative or irrational thoughts, attitudes, and core beliefs and how these impact his or her behaviors and thus his or her life. It is a very "problem-focused" form of therapy, meaning that the therapist's role is to aid the client in identifying and practicing strategies that will help achieve identified goals. In the case of less severe forms of depression, anxiety, and substance abuse, it has been found to be as effective as psychiatric medication. Indeed, for children and adolescents, CBT is recommended as the treatment of choice for many conditions, including depression, anxiety, and aggression.

> CBT asserts that thoughts and beliefs precede the emotions associated with unhealthy behaviors such as self-injury, substance abuse, relationship difficulties, eating disorders, depression, and anxiety.

CBT asserts that it is thoughts and beliefs precede the emotions associated with unhealthy behaviors that drive negative behaviors such as self-injury, substance abuse, relationship difficulties, eating disorders, depression, and anxiety. CBT works by helping clients to identify "automatic thoughts"—thoughts or images that are so familiar and come to mind seemingly automatically in response to an event—and patterns in these automatic thoughts that can lead to distorted thinking, called "cognitive distortions." Here are a few examples of common automatic thought patterns and cognitive distortions that we have all experienced (we will come back to these in a later chapter):

- *Personalizing*: Taking something personally when there is no evidence for this interpretation. For instance, interpreting someone's rough tone as them being annoyed with you.
- *Mindreading*: Guessing what someone is thinking when that might not be the case at all.
- *Catastrophizing*: Interpreting an unpleasant occurrence as a catastrophe.
- *Biased recall of social encounters*: A negative bias toward remembering negatives and not remembering the positives of a social situation.
- *Too many "shoulds" and "musts"*: These are dangerous little words, as these "rules" (e.g., "I must complete my to-do list every day") mean that we set unreasonably high expectations for ourselves that lead to feeling like failures.
- *Black-or-white thinking*: "If I don't get all As, then I'm a complete failure."

An individual's core beliefs, automatic thoughts, and cognitive distortions are often unconsciously linked to self-injury (or other maladaptive behaviors). Not surprisingly, self-criticism and layers of negative beliefs, assumptions, and automatic thoughts are common among those who self-injure. For instance, a teenager who feels rejected in a social situation at school may feel pain and anger in reaction to this, with an automatic thought of "I need to do something! I need to cut." A cognitive-behavioral therapist would help the teen to not only identify the thoughts that result from the social rejection, but would also help him to look for the core beliefs (in this case, thinking to himself, "it will always be this way" and "I'm no good; who would want to be friends with me?!") that are driving the immediate thoughts and feelings, as well as the cognitive distortions that need to be altered (black-or-white thinking; catastrophizing).

A CBT-trained therapist would work with a client to recognize these thoughts, question them, and then use other, healthier thoughts and beliefs to "reframe" the situation and allow the client to deal with uncomfortable feelings that arise as a result. There are a number of CBT strategies, but all of them include a series of questions and exercises intended to identify, challenge, and reframe core beliefs and narratives. These all aim to break the association between the negative thought and the associated narrative. The intense negative emotions generated by the thoughts are often diminished, along with the need for relief through self-injury. CBT-focused therapists also work with their clients to strengthen healthy skills for coping, communicating, and solving problems.

While most clients catch on to CBT techniques fairly easily and can use them outside of the therapist's office, it's not uncommon in the beginning to have clients explain that their self-injury "just happens" and that there are no identifiable thoughts or feelings leading up to or following the self-injury. A skilled cognitive therapist will use respectful questions meant to aid in bringing these largely hidden beliefs, assumptions, or thoughts and the resulting feelings to the surface.

As you might imagine, episodes of self-injury are commonly associated with thoughts of self-criticism and pessimistic attitudes and beliefs. These might include deep beliefs related to incompetence and lovability or that emotional pain is somehow deserved as punishment. Thoughts such as "I can't tolerate this, I need to *do* something" are common and often lead to feelings of sadness and panic. Alternatively, thoughts such as "self-injury is the quickest way to make this pain go away" can lead to feelings of relief in the anticipation of the physiological response and release of pain that tends to accompany self-injury for many chronic users. We'll discuss more of these cognitive strategies and how you can help your teen and yourself in Section 4. In the meantime, we have included at the end of this chapter an Automatic Thoughts Record that we would encourage you to fill out for yourself and possibly work on with your teen to get started with keeping track of situations that trigger self-injury thoughts or behavior and the associated thoughts and emotions.

Does it work? CBT has been shown to be effective in treating a diverse array of problems, ranging from anxiety and depression to schizophrenia and suicidal thoughts. Adults, teenagers, and children have benefited from these strategies. For instance, interesting work has been done by psychologist Philip Kendall and colleagues providing CBT to children and teens with anxiety disorders, with those receiving 16 weeks of CBT showing tremendous gains and many returning to within normal levels of anxiety as compared to those who had not received treatment.[8] Indeed, the benefits of CBT are many, particularly since it consists of fairly simple techniques and is easy to learn for most people. Moreover, it is typically delivered over the short term and is fairly cost-effective.

Most research studies examining the effectiveness of CBT intervention for suicidal and nonsuicidal thoughts and behaviors include a family component. Indeed, those studies examining CBT delivered only to the teenager (with no parent support) were found to do no better than therapy that simply consists of providing emotional support and encouragement.[9] This finding underscores the value of relationships and their importance in therapy. The family component of CBT often focuses on family skills training in the areas of problem-solving and communication. In addition to meeting with the teen alone, the CBT therapist would also meet regularly with the teen, parents, and any other family members to sort through issues raised in the teen's sessions, aid the family in developing new skills for working with one another, and develop some specific steps that families could work toward at home as "homework" in between therapy sessions.

> The family component of CBT often focuses on family skills training in the areas of problem-solving and communication.

An example of this approach is described well by Christianne Esposito-Smythers and colleagues in a form of therapy called *integrated CBT* (I-CBT), a method that utilizes a variety of individual CBT sessions, family CBT, and parent training sessions. In their study, adolescents who had recently attempted suicide or were seriously contemplating suicide and who had high levels of depression and substance abuse difficulties received either this specialized I-CBT treatment provided by specially trained counselors or a traditional psychotherapy provided by counselors in the community (as noted earlier, this is referred to as "treatment as usual").[10] Families receiving I-CBT met weekly for the first 6 months of therapy, followed by biweekly sessions for 3 months, and then monthly for 3 months. An option for medication was provided to those in either condition who were in need and was delivered free of charge. Over the course of treatment and at follow-up 1 year later, teens enrolled in the I-CBT showed significant reductions in suicide attempts (5% in I-CBT vs. 35% traditional therapy), as well as fewer emergency department visits and inpatient psychiatric hospitalizations. By 18 months, only 7% of I-CBT participants had a depressive disorder, while 31% of traditional therapy participants still met criteria for a depressive disorder. Teens receiving I-CBT also reported less alcohol and marijuana use throughout treatment. This is particularly important, as we know that substance use and abuse increase the risk for suicidal behavior among teens. An important takeaway message from this research is that the CBT skills and techniques learned in individual therapy are most beneficial when they are comprehensively delivered to teen, parents, and family, so that there are many opportunities for skills training and practice in developing these new ways of thinking. While self-injury behaviors were not looked at specifically in this study, nearly three-quarters of the participants reported a history of self-injury before starting the treatment, and reductions in the other behavior areas do suggest that there were likely to be reductions in NSSI as well.[11]

Dialectical Behavior Therapy

What is it and how does it work? Dialectical behavior therapy (DBT) was one of the first treatments to specifically target self-harm (suicidal and nonsuicidal) thoughts and behaviors. Originally designed to treat adult patients with borderline personality disorder, it has since been modified for adolescents with a history of self-harm. Developed by Marsha Linehan, DBT has roots in both CBT and Zen Buddhism.[12] It adds to the previously described CBT approach an additional focus on regulating emotions. From the perspective of DBT, many problematic teen behaviors (such as suicidal and NSSI behaviors) can be explained by difficulties with self-regulating the *internal emotional landscape* (as well as thoughts, as described earlier). This can lead to difficulty managing interpersonal conflicts and a low ability to tolerate difficult emotions or stress. Much of what is done in DBT emphasizes teaching skills for using balanced thinking, feeling, and acting, derived from the Buddhist idea of "walking the middle path." Using enhanced self-awareness and discipline to self-regulate, developing the ability to take different perspectives and resolve conflict, and being able to accept and tolerate emotional discomfort are the key strategies taught.

DBT commonly includes weekly individual therapy, weekly group skills training, and skills coaching by phone with the therapist as needed. For adolescents, when feasible, group skills training can take the form of multifamily skills groups, in which several parents and their teens learn the same content side by side, with the teens offering support and modeling coping strategies for one another. Separate parenting and family sessions may also be appropriate. As one mother describes,

> We began DBT both as a family and individually for [my] child. This has been tremendously helpful to her to gain insight and offer her behavior alternatives.
>
> —*Megan, on value of DBT for her child and family*

This form of DBT is, unsurprisingly, potentially the most time-consuming of the psychotherapy treatments for self-injury, typically lasting about 1 year.

Does it work? Research does support the use of DBT in the treatment of suicidal and NSSI behaviors.[13] Among adult women, a course of 6 months of DBT has been shown to decrease self-injury behaviors and urges. Less is known about the effectiveness of DBT with adolescents who self-injure, although several small studies (sample sizes ranged from 12 to 25 adolescents) have examined 6- to 12-month DBT interventions in adolescents and found significant reductions in suicidal and NSSI behaviors.[14] Other work has compared a 12-week DBT intervention with a more generic, supportive therapy and found that fewer adolescents attempted suicide in the DBT group than did those receiving the comparison supportive therapy group. Those teens receiving DBT also reported significantly fewer suicidal thoughts at the end of treatment.[15] What is missing from research exploring the effectiveness of DBT in adolescents is a study that compares year-long DBT treatment (the way that it is commonly delivered in outpatient settings) with a less intensive, standard supportive therapy that is more commonly delivered in community mental health settings.[16]

Despite what we do not know, DBT currently has the most scientific support for reducing self-harm behaviors. It may not, however, be for everyone. It typically involves intensive—sometimes inpatient—treatment ranging from 3 months to 1 year. A typical DBT psychotherapy intervention may not be practical with respect

DBT currently has the most scientific support for reducing self-harm behaviors.

to cost and availability of resources. Further, DBT may be more intensive than necessary for reducing self-injury in individuals who do not have a long-standing history of engaging in self-harm or other mental health challenges. Indeed, Barent Walsh, a well-respected clinician and author of several books on treating self-injury, describes DBT as a complex, intensive, and comprehensive treatment used with clients who have complex histories of self-harm behaviors.

A brief form of DBT designed specifically for treating self-injury has been developed by psychologist Margaret Andover. This treatment (abbreviated T-SIB) combines CBT and DBT techniques.[17] Consisting of nine weekly individual sessions lasting 1 hour each, it involves educating clients about self-injury, addressing the pros and cons of behavior change, identifying possible triggers and consequences of self-harm behaviors and urges, and finding alternatives to self-harm. Additional issues are targeted on an as-needed basis with three additional topic areas that cover interpersonal communication, cognitive distortions, and distress tolerance. The results are promising, with decreases at post-treatment in depression levels, number of days and episodes of self-injury, and reduced urges to self-injure. More than 75% of participants reported at least a 50% reduction in the number of self-injury episodes. This is particularly meaningful given the short length of treatment. Nevertheless, while results from this new work are promising, there is still much to be learned, such as whether improvements from therapy are seen over the long term and whether this treatment does as well as other existing treatments available for NSSI.

Problem-Solving Therapy

What is it and how does it work? As you might imagine, research suggests that individuals who engage in self-injury often have poor problem-solving skills and have difficulty thinking of alternative ways of managing problem situations. Problem-solving therapy (PST) is intended to help clients identify and solve problems that they encounter in their lives and teach healthy coping and problem-solving skills that allow for dealing more effectively with issues they encounter in the future.[18] In PST, the client typically meets with the therapist individually, although sometimes therapy can involve family members and group meetings. PST involves teaching a series of problem-solving steps such as problem identification and goal setting, brainstorming and assessing possible solutions, identifying and implementing a solution, and evaluating its success. PST is often combined with elements of cognitive, interpersonal, and behavioral therapy to improve effectiveness and can be used in FBT as well. One example of this is a very structured form of therapy in which a therapist delivers six sessions of therapy as it is laid out in a therapy manual. *Manual-assisted cognitive-behavioral therapy* (MACT) was developed to explicitly target self-harm urges and behaviors.[19] The six sessions consist of short-term problem-solving and CBT intervention that can be used in addition to existing therapy one may be receiving. The benefit of having these structured six sessions laid out in a therapy manual is their ease of use for both the client and the therapist.

> PST involves teaching a series of problem-solving steps such as problem identification and goal setting, brainstorming and assessing possible solutions, identifying and implementing a solution, and evaluating its success.

Does it work? Several RCTs have been conducted to evaluate the effectiveness of MACT in reducing self-injury in adults (although not teens, as of yet). In general, participants who received MACT reported significantly fewer self-injury episodes (even up to 12 months later). Other studies have also found improvements in suicidal ideation, hopelessness, and depression symptoms.[20] Overall, while studies do suggest that PST, particularly when combined with other CBT therapy skills, shows promise for reducing self-injury, studies to date have largely focused on adults, and additional research is needed to explore use of MACT among teenagers.

Intensive Outpatient and Residential Treatment Programs

Thus far we have been describing therapies used in both outpatient (i.e., not residential) and hospital settings. By its very nature, outpatient therapy is designed to assist those patients who are not at immediate risk of harming themselves or others. For those who may require more intensive treatment, who are at risk of severely injuring themselves, have serious mental illness, or do not have access to other outpatient therapies, various forms of intensive residential treatment programs are available. These run a wide gamut and include intensive inpatient hospital programs, day hospital and intensive outpatient programs, and community-based group homes or special residential schools. For a more thorough description of these various types of programs, consult Michael Hollander's book, *Helping Teens Who Cut.*[21]

While the programs themselves may differ in their structure, setting, and how much therapy is provided, these are all considered intensive programs because they involve a teenager spending much of his or her daytime hours, if not 24 hours, under professional care. Unfortunately, however, there is very little research that has evaluated which of these programs are effective and for whom. While these services are not suitable for everyone, there is clearly a need for these types of services during critical times. As one father indicated:

> Intensive outpatient therapy taught us both how to talk to each other. I saw my part and was helped to change in order to parent my daughter toward what she needed
>   —*Bruno, on the value of therapy in improving family relations*

Does My Child Need Intensive Therapy?

Intensive therapies such as those just discussed are typically reserved for people who are either currently in crisis or have a long history of mental health difficulties with little improvement from traditional therapies (such as weekly counseling appointments). If you believe that your child is in imminent, life-threatening danger, your first step would be to seek immediate assistance from emergency personnel. Emergency Department staff will be able to evaluate your child and her situation to determine whether she may benefit from admission to an inpatient facility to help stabilize her. They can also provide referrals and community mental health resources for you and your family. For those who are connected to a mental health provider already, we encourage you to speak with them about what they believe are important indicators of whether more intensive therapy is warranted. This might involve more intensive or frequent psychotherapy or perhaps the addition of medication.

Psychopharmacological Treatment for Self-Injury

Most parents wonder about the use of medications in the treatment of self-injury. Can medications be helpful to your child? What symptoms are they aimed at treating? Are there risks associated with taking these medications?

To be clear, we are learning more each year about how to effectively use psychological therapies and techniques to treat self-injury. Indeed, studies to date indicate that behavioral interventions (as described earlier) are more likely to reduce self-injury in the short term than are pharmacological interventions.[22] Unfortunately, the same cannot be said for our understanding of the role of the brain, medications, and their effect on self-injury. We understand some of the basic neural associations, but we do not yet know how to modify neural processes to alter self-injury behaviors. In other words, scientists do not yet know what medications work well for managing self-injury. Unfortunately, there are very few studies evaluating the use of medications for the treatment of NSSI in adults or adolescents, so decisions are often made on a case-by-case basis among a psychiatrist, teen, and parents.

> Studies to date indicate that behavioral interventions are more likely to reduce self-injury in the short term than are pharmacological interventions.

Looking for a "magic bullet" of sorts, parents are often surprised to learn that there is *no* medication devoted specifically to the treatment of self-injury. Medications can be prescribed by psychiatrists for teens who are experiencing other commonly occurring symptoms, such as depression or anxiety. For instance, research suggests there is a high prevalence of depression among individuals who self-injure. In these cases, the use of antidepressant medications, such as fluoxetine (Prozac), sertraline (Zoloft), paroxetine (Paxil), citalopram (Celexa), and escitalopram (Lexapro) (a class of drugs known as *selective-serotonin reuptake inhibitors* or SSRIs), has been shown to reduce depressive symptoms as well as to decrease self-injury *among some individuals.*[23]

In some individuals who self-injure, anxiety can also be present. In these cases, some psychiatrists may recommend the use of antianxiety medications, such as lorazepam (Ativan) or diazepam (Valium) (a class of drugs known as benzodiazepines). Unfortunately, results are mixed in the effectiveness of these medications, with some patients with self-injury and anxiety benefiting, while others become worse with benzodiazepine treatment.

Mood stabilizers, such as valproate or lithium carbonate, may be appropriate when wildly fluctuating mood is an issue, as is the case with a diagnosis of bipolar disorder. These have not been shown to be effective for treating self-injury when there are no signs of mood fluctuations also occurring, and there are potentially serious side effects involved in their use, including an increased risk of suicide.

While less common, if psychotic symptoms such as delusions or hallucinations are present, then a psychiatrist may recommend a trial of an atypical antipsychotic medication (such as aripiprazole and ziprasidone). For instance, among adults with borderline personality disorder, one RCT found that more participants were likely to abstain from self-injury during treatment with aripiprazole and at the 18-month follow-up compared with those receiving a placebo.[24]

What this information should suggest is a clear need for a detailed, focused assessment of the self-injuring youth before any decisions are made about pursuing medication. Your child's pediatrician or therapist can assist with providing recommendations for a psychiatrist who can evaluate your child's situation.[25]

We provide here a list of important things for the psychiatrist to consider in assessing whether medication may be appropriate for your child:

- Evaluation of your child's current behavior patterns and under what circumstances the self-injury occurs; if you or your child has kept a journal that documents when self-injury has occurred and under what circumstances, this can be useful information to provide.

- Any additional psychological symptoms that your child may be experiencing or clinical diagnoses he or she may have received, such as depression, stress or anxiety, or other behavioral difficulties, such as issues with peers.
- Current and historical life context, including the role of home, school, and peer environments. Have there been any changes in behavior at home or at school? Have grades gone down? Is your child more isolated than usual or hanging with a different crowd? Has there been any upheaval recently in the family?

The assessment process helps to identify developmental, social, interpersonal, and historical factors that may be contributing to the self-injury and what might be the best possible route for therapy. Whether psychological therapy, medication, or a combination of the two is recommended, it remains critical that assessment continues throughout treatment in order to evaluate both improvements and any setbacks experienced.

Activities

Activity 1: *The Automatic Thoughts Record: A Helpful First Step for Understanding Triggers for Self-Injury*

As discussed in this chapter, most psychological therapies for self-injury target the vicious cycle of situations, thoughts, and emotions that contribute to and/or are a result of self-injury. Doing this well takes some patience and practice, but it can offer valuable information that will help to change unhealthy, negative behavior patterns. It is common for people to initially express doubt that this technique will work for them. They may say things like, "How can this possibly help me to feel better?" or they otherwise express disbelief that it is possible to change their moods or how they think about something at all.

Here you'll find the first steps in what is called an Automatic Thoughts Record. We'll discuss this more in the last section of this book, adding on additional pieces of information that will help you to alter the way you're thinking and reacting to trigger situations.

A sample Automatic Thoughts Record is presented here, partially filled out with an example. Additional spaces are provided below this example for you to begin your own reflections and observations. You may find it helpful to record these thoughts as they come up and the feelings that you have as a result of them. Note that this does take some practice. Don't give up! Sometimes you may find it easiest to start with the feeling(s) that you're experiencing, then backtrack to try and understand what thought you might have had that caused you to feel that way. We will expand on this technique more in Section 3, but please know that the more you can observe and record your thoughts and feelings now, the easier it will be to work to change some of those negative thoughts and also help your teen to develop and use these skills.

While the examples provided in this Automatic Thoughts Record target experiences parents may have, there is no reason that your child wouldn't benefit from considering these steps and how situations are tied to his thoughts and feelings. If he is interested and willing to keep a journal and record these connections, this information might provide valuable insight to him—and perhaps assist in conversations he may have with a therapist. However, if he is not willing at present to keep track of these connections, that is all right, too.

Automatic Thoughts Record

When you notice a change in your mood, ask yourself, "What's going through my mind right now?"

Date/ Time	Situation	Automatic Thought	Emotion(s)
	What led to the change in your mood? What distressing physical sensations did you experience?	What thoughts or images went through your mind? On a scale from 0–100, how much did you believe them at the time?	What emotions did you feel at the time? On a scale from 0–100, how intense was the emotion?
Friday, 11/4, 5 pm	Noticed new cuts on my child's wrist	"She's never going to get better; she's out of control" "I am heartbroken" "What is wrong with our family?!"	Anxiety, guilt, fear, anger
Tuesday, 11/8, 3:30 pm	My child threatened to cut again if I did not do what he wanted	"He is manipulating me"	Anger, anxiety

Activity 2: What's Your Mindset?

A quiz for parents and children to take separately before proceeding to Chapter 8.

Parent Quiz

For the 20 questions given here, please rate each on whether you strongly disagree to strongly agree. Once you and your child have each taken this quiz, feel free to score them and share your responses with one another.

	Strongly disagree	Slightly disagree	Slightly agree	Strongly agree
1. Intelligence is something people are born with that can't be changed.				
2. No matter how capable you are, there are always new things to learn.				
3. You can substantially change how smart you are.				
4. You are a certain kind of person, and there is not much that can be done to really change that.				
5. You can always change basic things about the kind of person you are.				
6. Talents can be learned by anyone.				

	Strongly disagree	Slightly disagree	Slightly agree	Strongly agree
7. Only a few people will be truly good at a particular talent—you have to be "born with it."				
8. Parenting comes more naturally for mothers than for fathers.				
9. The harder you work at something, the better you will be at it.				
10. No matter what kind of person you are, you can always change substantially.				
11. Trying new things is stressful for me and I avoid it.				
12. Some people are good and kind, and some are not—it's not often that people change.				
13. I appreciate when people (such as parents, coaches, teachers) give me feedback about my performance.				

	Strongly disagree	Slightly disagree	Slightly agree	Strongly agree
14. I often get angry when I get negative feedback about my performance.				
15. All human beings are capable of learning.				
16. You can learn new things, but you can't really change how smart you are.				
17. You can do things differently, but the important parts of who you are can't really be changed.				
18. Human beings are basically good, but sometimes make terrible decisions.				
19. I like to learn new things.				
20. Truly smart people do not need to try hard.				

Youth Quiz

For the 20 questions given here, please rate each on whether you strongly disagree to strongly agree.

	Strongly disagree	Slightly disagree	Slightly agree	Strongly agree
1. Intelligence is something people are born with that can't be changed.				
2. No matter how capable you are, there are always new things to learn.				
3. You can substantially change how smart you are.				
4. You are a certain kind of person, and there is not much that can be done to really change that.				
5. You can always change basic things about the kind of person you are.				
6. Talents can be learned by anyone.				
7. Only a few people will be truly good at a particular talent—you have to be "born with it."				

	Strongly disagree	Slightly disagree	Slightly agree	Strongly agree
8. Parenting comes more naturally for mothers than for fathers.				
9. The harder you work at something, the better you will be at it.				
10. No matter what kind of person you are, you can always change substantially.				
11. Trying new things is stressful for me and I avoid it.				
12. Some people are good and kind, and some are not—it's not often that people change.				
13. I appreciate when people (such as parents, coaches, teachers) give me feedback about my performance.				
14. I often get angry when I get negative feedback about my performance.				

	Strongly disagree	Slightly disagree	Slightly agree	Strongly agree
15. All human beings are capable of learning.				
16. You can learn new things, but you can't really change how smart you are.				
17. You can do things differently, but the important parts of who you are can't really be changed.				
18. Human beings are basically good, but sometimes make terrible decisions.				
19. I like to learn new things.				
20. Truly smart people do not need to try hard.				

Adapted from http://www.classroom20.com/forum/topics/motivating-students-with

What's Your Mindset: Scoring

Growth mindset questions are items #2, 3, 5, 6, 9, 10, 13, 15, 18, and 19. Each of these responses is scored in the following way:

Strongly agree = 3 points
Agree = 2 points
Disagree = 1 point
Strongly disagree = 0 points
Growth score:_____

Fixed mindset questions are items #1, 4, 7, 8, 11, 12, 14, 16, 17, and 20. Each of these responses is scored in the following way:

Strongly agree = 0 points
Agree = 1 points
Disagree = 2 point
Strongly disagree = 3 points
Fixed score:_____

How did you do? Add up your Growth score and your Fixed score for your total score:_____.

Here's what it means:

45–60 points = Strong Growth Mindset
34–44 points = Growth Mindset with some Fixed ideas
21–33 points = Fixed Mindset with some Growth ideas
0–20 points = Strong Fixed Mindset

This quiz measures beliefs about what is termed the "fixed" versus "growth" continuum of mindset. The idea behind this continuum is that it is our *belief* about whether change is or is not possible that most predicts whether change happens. Psychologist Carol Dweck and her colleagues, for example, studied several hundred young women at a university to understand how their mindsets influenced their performance in math and their desire to pursue math. They found that the extent to which women believed that math ability was fixed or changeable strongly predicted their performance in math as well as their desire to pursue it.

In other words, people with a *fixed mindset* tend to believe that core abilities and/or traits are inherited and generally unchangeable. Those with a fixed mindset orientation believe that only limited change is possible or expected. The best one can do in this case is to endure the difficulty that comes with running up against the limits of one's own natural ability, character, or external circumstances. Doing one's best to avoid or get past life's challenges, then, becomes a primary goal of individuals with fixed mindsets. Change can feel totally impossible in these cases.

People with a *growth mindset*, on the other hand, tend to see ability and character traits as qualities that can be developed or altered through effort and discipline. They believe that effort is needed to change—sometimes a lot of effort—but that change is inherently possible. This kind of mindset tends to result in a person having a high degree of curiosity and a "let's figure this out" orientation. We talk more about growth and fixed mindsets in Chapter 8.

Beyond Surviving

From Disorder to Growth and Discovery

I'm thankful that I went through it. I know that sounds kind of crazy but I learned so much about myself and how to break down all those layers and find who it is I really am and, in the process trying out a thousand different masks, personalities, clothes, everything that comes along with it. For me it is that I was given a chance to love myself and to really prove that this life is worth it. Every step I take since then is huge leaps and it's just beautiful; where I am now is only because I went through all of that. So, in a lot of ways I needed to go through all that. And it was terrible and I would never do it again and I would never want anyone to go through that. But to have gone through something so dark and bad is . . . like how deep I was in that is as deep as I am now and happiness. It's awesome.

—Rachel, 19 years, reflections on her self-injury

S TOPPING SELF-INJURY IS OFTEN THE GOAL THAT parents and, in some cases, clinicians will use to gauge progress and/or enhanced well-being. This makes sense since it is the behavior that causes so much pain in those who witness it and in the person who uses it. But a growing body of research supports the idea that, in addition to the stress they cause, adversity and trauma can also lead to personal growth.[1] Moreover, feeling optimistic and/or expectant that growth can occur as a result of challenges has been linked to well-being in a variety of areas. We see this process at work in nonsuicidal self-injury (NSSI) as well.

For many, the process of changing self-injury behavior can be a powerful growth opportunity—one that ushers in greater self-understanding and self-compassion. As Rachel's words demonstrate, it is possible to do more than merely survive the experience. In the process of figuring out how one arrived at wanting or needing to self-injure, it is not uncommon to experience a cascade of realizations and changes in outlook, attitude, effort, and discipline that lead to more than quitting self-injury. And it can do this for more than the person in your family who self-injures—it can affect multiple members of the family or the whole family system.

In two recent studies we conducted, we aimed to figure out how often growth happens as a result of having gone through a period of self-injury. First, we found that about a third of people who had engaged in chronic self-injury as a way of coping reported psychological growth as a result of the experience.[2] In this study, "growth" was defined by a scale which measured the extent to which respondents believed that the experience of self-injury promoted greater emotional or psychological self-awareness, a desire to help others, and more honest conversations with other people in their lives. Growth was predicted by strong connections to others, willingness to confide in one or more people honestly, and having come face to face with questions about the value and meaning of one's life.

> For many, the process of changing self-injury behavior can be a powerful growth opportunity—one that ushers in greater self-understanding and self-compassion.

In the second study, we asked parents of individuals who self-injure[3] to reflect on how hopeful they were that their child would grow as a result of having self-injured. We also wanted to learn how hopeful parents themselves were that *they personally* would grow as a result of having a self-injurious child. Of the 169 parents who participated, most of whom had children with multiple mental health challenges, more than a quarter felt that having a child who struggled with self-injury had brought them closer and another quarter felt that, although their child's self-injury experience had pushed them apart, they were confident that the relationship would recover. Only 15% perceived that the self-injury had pushed them apart and left them uncertain about whether they would recover. Notably, 51% indicated that they were very optimistic that their child would experience personal growth as a result of their experience, and 53% of all parents said that they were very optimistic about their own growth. Comments such as these were common:

> My child and I now allow each other to be human, to say, "I am sorry" and to forgive each other for not being "perfect." She knows she is loved and supported and has voiced that to all of her therapists.
>
> She is more in tune with her feelings, better able to voice them, and better able to be OK with whatever a person's response might be.
>
> I have learned so much about myself, my parenting style, my marriage and my children because self-injury entered our lives. It has made me more introspective about what she needs from a parent to be healthy.
>
> Seeing how she is able to accept herself now. Seeing those things translate into a much more socially outgoing child who has developed very close loving relationships with friends and family.

What is interesting and important to note is that growth tends to happen when one is open to growing or seeing that there is value even when things are very hard. *Growth is more a mindset than it is a set of behaviors.* Studies of the behavior change process, regardless of the behavior one is trying to change, consistently show that while we tend to think about behavior change as primarily a matter of deciding to stop particular behaviors and then having the willpower to "just do it," it simply does not work that way. A person is most likely to be successful in stopping a deeply ingrained negative habit, such as self-injury, when she also finds inspiration, meaning, and purpose in what she has experienced or comes to better understand her relationship to the behavior. As Tonya puts it:

I was able to stop when I quit thinking that I just had to leave it behind altogether. It was when I understood that it had been teaching
me that I needed to learn to ask for help and to respect the pull it had
on me that I was really able to stop.
　　　　　　—*Tonya, 23, on how she finally stopped self-injuring*

How Do We Do More Than Survive This? The Growth-Oriented Mindset

Why is it that some people who experience a hard period of life, like self-injury, look back and say, "Ah, that was horrible, I don't ever want to think about it. I don't want to deal with it. I don't want to talk about it," while others look back and say, "It was really hard, but I learned a lot about myself. I now have insight I did not have and I feel stronger and more capable of helping myself and others than ever before"? One of the most fascinating trends we notice in the healing process is that, even though stopping self-injury is one thing everyone who has stopped has in common, the similarities often end there. While many who successfully stop injuring talk about being relieved that self-injury is in their past and are intent on not revisiting it, others are grateful that they had the experience because they or their families grew so much stronger and/or closer.

How does this happen? In a very robust and long-standing line of study, psychologist Carol Dweck has repeatedly demonstrated that life success, in tangible (material success) and intangible (emotional and relational well-being and connection) ways, can be traced to what she calls "mindsets."[4] A mindset is basically one or more beliefs we each carry around about ourselves and our most essential qualities. We all have mindsets, though few of us take time to figure out what these are and to see how our mindsets subtly and overtly shape our views of the world, our behaviors, and our interactions with others.

One dimension of mindsets relates to how we view qualities such as intelligence, personality, and talents. If you and your child took the "What's Your Mindset?" quiz at the end of the previous chapter, then you can use the following to help with interpreting your scores.

Growth-Oriented Mindset and Parenting

What does this have to do with parenting? It turns out that having a fixed versus growth mindset orientation does not simply predict how we see ourselves or how hard we are willing to work to change things, but it also influences what we assume about others' capacities as well. For example, teachers with a growth-oriented mindset are much more likely to challenge students in a way that leads them to produce higher quality work, and the students in turn work harder and perform better.[5] In contrast, teachers with a fixed mindset toward personal ability and character will tend to form ideas around children based on their test scores, intelligence scores, or character traits that track students as low or high ability (e.g., "Johnny performed poorly on his fourth-grade standardized testing and therefore he likely doesn't have much academic ability, and minimal effort should be put into him")—sometimes for years.

Parents may not be quite so likely to develop these rigid notions of abilities and aptitudes with their own children, but parents do form opinions about their children's innate abilities or character capacities and limitations and then react to those in alignment with their own assumptions about how fixed or changeable these abilities are. Much of the time this is not terribly conscious. It can, however, have a very significant effect on how children will view their own abilities to grow or, alternatively, to be stuck. Parents' reactions to their children's self-injury and healing process are affected by whether they believe growth and change are possible for their children and/or their families as a whole.

The good news is that it is possible to alter a mindset once we become aware of our inherent mindset tendencies. Since parenting mindsets can significantly affect child outcomes, it is worth working on if you find that you are naturally more fixed in orientation. By looking at the responses you gave to the "What's Your Mindset" activity in the last chapter, you can get a feel for where you fall on the spectrum. In general, parents with a growth-oriented mindset are more easily able to recognize opportunities for increased closeness, communication, and/or authentic sharing even in the midst of difficult moments. This openness to communication tends to result in exchanges between parent and child that foster both enhanced closeness *and* greater resilience that will help with handling future challenges. Over time, what seem like small differences toward a growth orientation can lead to

> Growth-oriented mindsets are not about giving in, lowering expectations, or constantly validating your child's perceptions regardless of how skewed they seem to you. It is quite the opposite, in fact.

big changes in the outcomes for yourself and your child, as well as for the family system in general. It is important to note that growth-oriented mindsets are not about giving in, lowering expectations, or constantly validating your child's perceptions regardless of how skewed they seem to you. It is quite the opposite, in fact. Adopting a growth-oriented mindset means that you hold a realistic but hopeful vision of what you know your child can accomplish and that you regularly model your language and your actions to communicate that vision to your child.

The following reflection-based case study is from Shria, a parent whose 16-year-old child struggled for more than a year with multiple mental health challenges, including depression and thoughts of suicide. It is a good example of how using a growth-oriented mindset feels from a parent's perspective.

When my daughter was really struggling with depression, for a good chunk of her 11th-grade year, I had the opportunity to refine my capacity to find the subtle shifts that were happening and to respond to them in ways that I hoped would amplify their effect. I knew that she was really stuck in a pattern of negative thinking, feeling, and expectation and that this cycle was creating, or at least contributing to, many of the seriously challenging situations she found herself in. She would not, however, respond well to positive moods, opportunities, or comments about herself, her future, or possible remedies to her challenges. It was exceptionally frustrating to be around her.

My first job was to deeply acknowledge that I could not fix things for her. Nor could I act in her place when she found herself trapped in a chronic negative cycle. Although I felt helpless, particularly when it was so clear to me what she could do to change things, I worked hard on "letting go" of attachment to the thought that I had to make things different. This helped me to really focus on playing supporter rather than doer and backing off when she clearly needed to struggle on her own (note to other parents: 2 years later she thanked me for this)! Even though it runs counter to parenting instincts to protect, acknowledging our children's separateness from us and supporting their own unique journey in the world is a way of communicating something akin to "I know you can do it." It may be terrifying for everyone at the time, but such moments are the building blocks of resilience and self-confidence.

My second job was to watch for small opportunities to gently point out that there were other ways of interpreting or responding to situations that were likely to generate fewer negative feelings and beliefs. Instead of being so focused on her behaviors (or apathy), I watched for opportunities to offer reframes for the ways in which her interpretation of events led to a sense of injustice or wounds that deepened her depression. Once I could do this without needing her to take my advice or see my perspective, I noticed that she was more likely to incorporate some element of my perspective, even if in a very small way. So, for example, when her boyfriend at the time started posting pictures of himself with other girls along with hook-up stories and she cried that he was betraying her on purpose, I validated this feeling but also reminded her that he was young like she was, and was also learning about how to deal with hard situations. I suspected, I told her, that he would eventually learn how to cope with his feelings differently but that he was still figuring it all out.

Shria was able to validate her daughter's feelings and promote compassion and understanding because these emotions are inherently more likely to ease the negative feelings and thoughts that reinforce the depression and negative behaviors. Also, by not vilifying her daughter's ex-boyfriend, she leaned on the broad principle in growth-oriented frameworks that suggests that *all* people are capable of change and growth; this is another way of saying "even the most hard-off of us, like you may feel yourself to be, can grow and change in positive ways." Shria continues:

> One of the first small signs that things were moving in a positive direction were in the area I now think of as the "small surprises." These were moments in which I totally anticipated a particular reaction from her to a stressful situation—a relational challenge or logistical challenge or something that I knew was simply difficult for her and likely to lead to a blowup of some sort. As she started to change, she started to react in slightly different ways. Usually it was not a radical difference, but in a case where she would have quit something out of frustration on day one, she was willing to hang in there for a little

longer and complain a little less. She may have still ended up drop-
ping out, but it took longer and was less dramatic than in the past.

At first, these were just moments, here and there, among what
had come to be simply her dominant negative state of mind. Slowly,
however, these surprises stopped being so surprising. Once this ball
got rolling, I noticed more sizeable shifts in moods, expectations of
herself, the future, and others, and engagement in positive life activities. These came across in her texts to me, comments, level of activity
and engagement, connections with peers, the food she ate, exercise
patterns, and the other many ways that she moved through her day.
It was clear that she was in a very different place.

My job during all of this, I knew, was to acknowledge her progress,
even if it was very modest. At the same time, I didn't want her to feel
like I was watching her like a hawk all the time so I didn't always make
a big deal out of everything I noticed. Most often, especially early on,
I would just simply and quietly say something that could be translated
as, "I'm impressed at how well you dealt with that situation. I think that
the comment your boyfriend made on Facebook may have really upset
you a few weeks ago. I can tell by what you just said that you understand
his behavior differently now. I'm sure it feels good to not feel quite so
bad as you might have in the past about it." Since it was hard for her to
generate her own positive feelings and to receive positives from others,
I knew that I needed to capitalize on moments when she was more re-
ceptive and provide validation. I also knew that I was serving as a role
model for how and what she could learn to notice in herself.

The general formula that Shria is describing here is to let her
daughter know that she had noticed a change for the better and then
to reinforce the positive emotional consequence for her (e.g., saying
something along the lines of "I am sure that feels better than it did
when you were thinking about it differently or when you reacted the
way you tended to in the past"). Since so much of the process of deep
change requires learning new ways of thinking, feeling, relating, and
doing, it is helpful to see how these new ways work through somebody else's eyes. As Shria summarizes:

Today, 2 years later, she is a very different person in so many ways.
She still struggles with reacting more negatively than positively at
first, but quickly self-corrects. She is also much more aware of what
she needs to do to keep from getting in a deep funk, and she has
much, much more emotional stamina than ever. She now wants to

use her life energies to work in international public health so she can assist others. Those dark nights for her were really dark for me as well, but I knew that I needed to quietly stand guard over my vision of the adult woman she was becoming and not get wrapped up in my and her (or her father's) fears about what she was in the moment. It paid off! She even wrote me a letter of appreciation recently in which she thanked me for supporting her when she needed it and letting her figure it out on her own when I felt like she needed that experience. I cannot tell you how great it felt to know that holding the highest vision of who she was and could be, even when I felt totally helpless in so many other ways, really made a difference.

How to Recognize and Promote Growth

The secret of health for both mind and body is not to mourn for the past, not to worry about the future, or not to anticipate troubles, but to live in the present moment wisely and earnestly.
—The Buddha

At this time, you may believe that it is unrealistic to hope for something above and beyond having a healthy child who does not turn to self-injury or other negative coping strategies to regulate emotion. That is understandable. Fortunately, understanding and applying a growth-oriented mindset is useful for all of your parenting and personal goals, regardless of how grand or modest they may be.

Table 8.1 provides several examples of how the fixed and growth mindsets may work relative to self-injury. Can you find yourself or your situation in there? Feel free to use the blank spaces at the bottom of the table to identify a situation you find yourself in and what you think the fixed- and growth-oriented mindset responses may be. It may also be helpful to place a star next to any situation you are experiencing that you would like to approach with a growth-mindset orientation. Having clear growth-mindset parenting goals will help you practice new ways of thinking and responding. Remember that everything you learn, practice, do, say, or in some way communicate in the presence of your child, even if not directed at him, models new ways of behavior for your child. In this way, your growth may also increase the likelihood of your child's growth.

Table 8.1 Fixed versus Growth Mindsets in Parenting a
    Self-injurious Child

Fixed mindset	Your situation	Growth mindset
My child is stuck, oversensitive, and/ or failing.	Interpreting your child's current state	My child is learning how to deal with the gift and challenge of sensing and feeling emotions intensely.
I/we hurt her by not being there for her or by <fill in the blank>. It is my/our fault.	How did you, your child, your family arrive here?	We have had some hard times in the past. All people have hard times. I wish it had not been this way, but learning how to deal with disappointment and/ or hurt can make my child (and me) stronger and more compassionate toward others.
My child cuts herself because she cannot cope with feelings. She is weak.	What her acting out (self-injury) behavior means	My child cuts herself to temporarily feel better and regroup. While it won't work well in the long run, I know she is working hard to deal with feelings she does not yet know how to deal with differently. I trust she will sometime.
My child is angry and hostile all of the time. He is just that way and will probably never change.	What your child's negative comments about you, herself, or others means about him	My child is afraid of the situations he is in and the emotions that they bring up. He is young and learning how to cope with things that seem overwhelming. This is going to be hard for us all since his first reaction to stress is negative, but I know he can learn how to do it differently once he understand himself better.

Table 8.1 Continued

Fixed mindset	Your situation	Growth mindset
She is wasting her life and time. She is losing the opportunity she should be taking to build skills that will secure her future.	Forecasting the future	My child is facing an intense opportunity to build her self awareness, understanding, and emotional capacity. Since these are critical for every relationship she will ever have, personal or professional, and for making decisions that fit her life, taking time now to learn how to work with herself is very useful.
We have been doing this for so long, and she does not seem to be changing at all. I am giving up hope.	When progress feels slow or nonexistent	My child is moving at a pace that works for him. I do wish he was moving more quickly, but I know that I do not have control over that; this is his life. I need to focus on balancing realistic support of him with my own need to not feel trapped in his life choices so much.
I am trapped in this and cannot get out. I will never feel good again.	When parental stress becomes overwhelming	My child's situation or way of dealing with hard situations is wearing on me. It is time for me to figure out how to make more space and time for me to attend to taking care of myself. This will help me and will model what positive self-care looks like for my child. We'll be okay.

Important Steps to Adopting a Growth-Oriented Mindset

Now that you are familiar with the growth-oriented framework, there are a few concrete areas to focus on in thinking about adopting this focus more often.

- *Believe up*: If you can see the possibility for change and a good life for someone who is clearly struggling, it will be easier for him to see this, too. Optimism and broadened thinking are infectious and critical to modeling healthier ways of thinking about future possibilities.

- *Respect readiness to change*: As we discussed earlier, individual willingness and ability to change is heavily dependent on a person's readiness for change. Someone in the Moratorium phase, for example, will be completely unwilling and unprepared to think about changing her self-injury behavior. She may, however, be able to understand that it is not okay to attend school or other social functions with open wounds displayed and that talking to peers about the practice is problematic. Helping her understand why this is, in a respectful and nondemeaning way, is likely to achieve the goal of protecting others *and* keeping her engaged in the process. Individuals further along with the change process can be assisted in more direct and active ways.

- *Provide authentic feedback and productive observations*: Self-injury, like a lot of negative habits, often relies on some degree of cognitive and emotional rigidity. An individual who is cognitively or emotionally rigid has difficulty shifting easily from task to task or from the expression of one emotion to another. They are easily "stuck" and have difficulty experiencing a full range of emotions (e.g., happiness, sadness, anger) or shaking off certain emotions or thoughts. When this inflexibility shows up in a person's life, it can be difficult to work with and around—for everyone! Change relies on an increased self-awareness of patterns coupled with an intention to change them. Helping others see these inflexible parts of themselves can be a real gift, provided that insight is constructively offered in a positive manner. Likewise, helping people see the ways in which they are naturally or newly flexible is very powerful and an important part of personal growth.

- *Recognize and support other people in your child's life*: People who self-injure are a part of families, peer groups, schools, and other groups experiencing the same journey. These are often the places where support can be found. But it is also possible to be triggered by these settings and groups as well. To the extent that it is possible to positively engage or support the social systems within which they are embedded, it will benefit your child. We will talk more about developing collaborations in Chapter 13.

- *Help your child identify and reinforce successes:* As necessary and helpful as it is to study the triggers (events, situations, feelings that lead to an urge or action to self-injure), it is equally useful to study and reinforce your child's success at overcoming these potential triggers. In other words, to pay attention to the events or situations in which an urge to self-injure has been successfully avoided. Acknowledging and knowing this provides a reason to celebrate and build positive feelings that help prevent future slips. It also makes relying on those strengths easier in the future. Moreover, taking time to reflect on successes can help everyone see slips for what they are: temporary bumps along the road to healing.

- *Count your blessings*: Taking "count your blessings" one step further, a journal can be used for noticing and keeping track of opportunities to experience gratitude. This can be one way to help someone focus on positive aspects of life and to increase engagement in the behavior change process. Indeed, we find this to be such an important part of healthy, positive communications that we've included an activity meant to help identify those positives in your life and cultivate gratitude.

Return to Compassion for Yourself and Your Child

All the advice that we have to offer here is compiled from thousands of moments that have been lived and experienced by us and by the parents we have interviewed. Some of those moments were exceptional examples of the "Aha! I nailed it!" variety, while others were flaming examples of just the opposite, followed by the inevitable, "I guess I should have handled *that* differently." Sometimes when we read books like this we can end up feeling like we are simply not up to the challenge of holding all of this vital information in mind at once. We are not aiming here to develop perfect parents or to develop perfect children. We are not perfect parents! The fact is, though, that your child does not need lessons in how to be perfect because none of us is or ever will be. Your child needs lessons in how to be human—living with integrity, good intentions, openness, and a willingness to continually make amends or make things right when they get out of balance. In short, your job is to show your child what it means to be the best kind of messy human she can be. This makes space for the moments you say things that you later regret, the moments you don't say anything at all but wish you had, and the times in which there's just nothing hopeful or uplifting to lean on.

> Your job is to show your child what it means to be the best kind of messy human she can be.

A growing number of studies show that compassion and gratitude for the things that go right in life, even if they are very tiny, lead to increased well-being in a variety of measurable ways. If you can allow yourself to have messy moments, then it's easier to understand how your child may be experiencing the more difficult messiness of authentic living and to help your child know that change is the only thing we can count on. There will always be more opportunities for doing things differently.

Activities

Activity 1: Keeping a Gratitude Journal: Noticing the Positives and Growing Gratitude

> *Give thanks for a little and you will find a lot.*
>
> —Hausa Proverb

Studies suggest that simple acts of gratitude, such as writing in a gratitude journal one to three times a week, can lead to greater happiness and life satisfaction.[6] Gratitude journals are helpful in developing the ability to see the good in the things, people, and experiences around us. Keeping track of these often small things allows us to see them as gifts, which guards against taking any of them for granted. Keeping a gratitude journal also helps us to savor pleasant small moments and surprises. For this reason, don't rush yourself through this. Take the time to appreciate and value each of these gifts.

There's no right or wrong way to keep a gratitude journal— electronic or handwritten, it's what works for you. The goal is to record things for which you feel grateful. This might be 5 things on one day, 3 on another, or perhaps 10 on a different day. The more specific and detailed you can be, the better. For instance, "I'm grateful for my friends taking detailed notes in my classes when I was out sick from school on Tuesday" is more effective than "I'm grateful for my friends." The things you list can be small or large. Consider: What are you grateful for, and why? Could you imagine your life without this person or experience?

Here is an example of a gratitude journal entry. We encourage both parents and their children to try regularly writing in a gratitude journal. Find a regular time—perhaps just before bed or Sunday mornings when the house is still quiet—and commit to this regular time. One to three times per week is most useful for this type of journaling and has been found to be more effective even than keeping a daily journal. You can also choose to get creative, perhaps drawing a picture of what you are grateful for, taping concert tickets to a journal page to remind yourself of a special evening with friends, and more. It's your journal, meant to inspire and motivate you.

Gratitude Journal

Date/Time	What I'm grateful for . . .
Tuesday, May 30	1. Feeling strong as I walked the dog on a sunny, warm morning. 2. The kids—for making me laugh as they tried to teach me their ballet routine. 3. The tasty sandwich I had for lunch today.

Parents as Partners

Skills and Tools for Helping Yourself and

Your Child

9

I Have Feelings, Too!

Understanding the Role of Our Own
Automatic Thoughts and Reactions

If there is anything that we wish to change in the child, we should first examine it and see whether it is not something that could better be changed in ourselves.

—Carl Jung

Every one of us has experienced the realization that we are simply acting out of fear, desire, or want without questioning where these impulses come from and whether our actions are good for us and others in our lives. Our brains evolved to move fluidly from one thought or feeling to the next, often seamlessly. We call this *mindless* or *automatic* because it occurs without any conscious awareness or effort. It *just happens.*

Many of our behaviors are as mindless as our wandering thoughts. The rapid cascade of perceiving something in our environment to reacting to it is an important part of our survival instincts.[1] However, mindless thoughts and reactions are often not conscious, and, once they are in motion, they tend to be self-reinforcing, meaning that they may happen over and over again. Such thought–emotion–behavior cascades happen often for all of us and typically show up as negative moods, comments, or actions. When we are aware of the cascade and the set of associations set in motion, we can consciously check in with ourselves to be sure our reactions are, in fact, balanced and understandable. When we act out of instinctive impulses and associations, our reactions can appear or feel out of proportion or otherwise untethered to whatever is going on in the moment. This can add fuel to an already burning fire, and that is pretty much never helpful.

This idea of the thought–emotion–behavior cascade is not new. We talked about the role this process plays in your child's life in Chapter 4. But since these automatic thoughts, feelings, and behaviors are with us all, we want to use the next two chapters to focus on how automatic thoughts impact *your* life, particularly when it comes to being a parent. Parenting a teenager can be challenging in its own right, but as the parent of a child who self-injures, you may be more likely than other parents to find yourself in situations that trigger your automatic thought–emotion–behavior cascade. Understanding and using a few of the core principles of mindfulness can often help slow things down and provide parents with more options for staying balanced. One of the core skills in doing this is to become aware of your own inherent patterns and tendencies. And, since thoughts tend to drive the cycle, it is useful to start there.

> As the parent of a child who self-injures, you may be more likely than other parents to find yourself in situations that trigger your automatic thought–emotion–behavior cascade.

Becoming Aware of Thought Patterns

Thoughts are funny things. They can be fleeting or enduring, conscious or unconscious, spoken or unspoken. We don't often take time to wonder much about thoughts, unless they are strong and persistent. Even in this case, however, we rarely stop to wonder where a thought comes from or to ask ourselves if it is true. Most of us are simply accustomed to walking around with a certain number of stressful thoughts (e.g., our to-do lists, doubts about ourselves and our abilities, worry about others' actions and intentions). We bend our lives around them because they are a constant part of our inner thought landscape. Even if we recognize that our thoughts don't necessarily reflect reality, or at least reality as someone else might see it, most of us don't understand (or at least appreciate) the link between thoughts, feelings, and our actions. Nor do most of us understand that our own thinking patterns, even if never spoken out loud, are likely perceived by our children (and partners, and even friends who know us well).

Sometimes our thoughts are the proverbial tip of the iceberg, obscuring a bundle of other thoughts and feelings. Most often, these are connected to our most personal core beliefs, those deeply held underlying values we all hold about ourselves and how the world works. Most of our core beliefs go unnoticed and unchallenged for long periods of time. They do, however, strongly influence our emotions and behaviors toward ourselves and others in ways that we may be completely unaware of. They operate in the background, coloring our interpretations of day-to-day experiences (this process is also called "cognitive appraisal"). Some of us tend to have more positively flavored core beliefs (think of optimists, for example), while others of us tend to think and feel more negatively (such as pessimists).

No matter where you might fall on the optimist–pessimist continuum, virtually all of us possess subtly biased cognitive appraisal patterns that favor negative interpretations. Psychologists call these *cognitive distortions*, or *automatic negative thoughts*, and they have deep evolutionary roots in helping humans defend themselves against potential sources of harm and buffer against disappointment.[2] The problem is that many of these patterns can shape our day-to-day and moment-to-moment communications and behaviors in ways that negatively impact our relationships. When working toward enhancing or changing family dynamics, as may be part of your goals, it is really helpful to be aware of what biases and distortions you may be bringing to the exchange. Even if it is uncomfortable to acknowledge our own biases, we all have more choice about how to interact with others when we understand our own patterns. Here, we describe common cognitive biases and examples of how they can color exchanges with a child.

What's Your Type? Common Cognitive Distortions

Cognitive distortions are tools our minds use to help us to make meaning of what we encounter outside of us (e.g., events, exchanges with others, or other kinds of stimuli). They are called *distortions* because the pattern of thinking we use in this state typically results in making us believe that something we think is true when it is, in fact, not true. They typically develop when we are young in response to repeated, or patterned, experiences. Since survival often depends on avoiding danger, negative experiences are especially "sticky," and our minds are quick to record key markers or red flags it can use in the future to detect and avoid similar negative experiences. After being formed, they tend to "run in the background," much like a computer program might—vigilant for patterns similar to those we have encountered before so they can defend us from feeling hurt or wounded.

While the mind creates these filters to create a sense of safety, these distortions often skew our ability to see and understand what is really going on *now*. They are basically forever responding to a set of past experiences. Unless we are very mindful and self-aware, cognitive distortions formed in childhood do not tend to mature as readily as our bodies do, so most adults continue to use distortions they formed as children.

When parents and children both have multiple or strong cognitive distortions in play, they can interact in ways that leave everyone feeling wounded and distant. We are all particularly vulnerable to cognitive distortions when we are feeling stressed or depressed, and parenting a child with chronic and sometimes unpredictable and disruptive behavior, such as self-injury, is more than enough to trigger distorted thinking. When cognitive distortions involve core beliefs about your self-injurious child or your relationship with your child, they can add a powerfully negative tone to the dynamic.

Are there specific types of cognitive distortions, you ask? Yes. Substantial research has been conducted in this area, and specialists have identified 10 of the most common cognitive distortions:

- Mental filtering
- Black and white thinking

- Overgeneralization
- Jumping to conclusions
- Catastrophizing
- Personalizing
- Blaming
- "Shoulds" and "musts"
- Fallacy of change
- Emotional reasoning

We all have cognitive distortions of one sort or another. Their type and the intensity with which we believe them can vary by context (e.g., when we're feeling tired vs. rested, relaxed vs. stressed) and/ or by person (e.g., a certain family member vs. best friend vs. co-worker). Since many of these thinking patterns are related, they may show up together and/or may change over time.

With practice, you can learn to recognize when you are engaging in one or more of these cognitive distortions and then use *mindfulness*, the practice of being present and moving out of the past, to consciously alter your thought patterns and/or your emotional/behavioral reactions. This can have a notable impact on the tone and outcome of the exchanges you have with your self-injurious child and other family members.

Cognitive Distortions in Action

Here, we describe the 10 common cognitive distortions, followed by real-life examples drawn from our work with families. Feel free to use the spaces provided to identify one or two examples of times you've noticed yourself engaging in these types of negative thinking patterns. If you cannot think of a time you have personally experienced one of these negative thought patterns, try to think of one in which you have observed another person engaging in the cognitive distortion.

1. **Mental filtering**: Mental filtering involves dwelling on the negative aspects of a situation, person, or setting while seriously minimizing or discounting altogether any positive aspects. Similarly, when positive qualities or accomplishments are presented, these are discounted.

Example: Whenever Bonnie talked about her daughter's self-injury to others, she spent most of the conversation describing how often her daughter relapses and makes life hard for the other children. She discounted any positive efforts her daughter was putting into changing her behaviors and life situation. Unfortunately, she had difficulty noting this same negative thought pattern in herself.

What Bonnie did: After noticing her pattern, Bonnie started an interaction journal in which she jotted down all of the negative things she noticed her daughter doing (this was easy!), but, for every negative entry she made, she forced herself to find at least one positive detail. While she found this a bit challenging at first, it became easier over time.

Example from your life:
Example you've observed in your child or other family member:

What could be done to change it:

2. **Black-and-white thinking**: This is most commonly framed as "all-or-nothing" thinking, or thinking in "black-and-white" terms. One is either all good or bad, right or wrong, perfect or imperfect—there is no middle ground. It is absolute. The problem with this, of course, is that life is mostly made up of complex situations—more shades of gray than black or white. We must learn to appreciate other perspectives and ways to interpret situations that we find ourselves in.

Example: Whenever she found out that Keesha had cut, Simone was quick to assume that Keesha had gone back to her old pattern. In Simone's mind, Keesha was either "giving herself" to her self-injury or totally "done" with self-injury, there was not much in between. Because of this, Simone's response to her daughter's self-injury was exaggerated and uneven.

What Simone did: As Simone began to recognize this pattern, she also began to see what a big effect her all-or-nothing mindset had on her emotions (extreme disappointment and feelings of betrayal if her daughter slipped or extreme relief when she thought, "whew, it is over and now we can go back to normal"). Whenever she found herself in one or the other space, she would tell herself "it is not all wrong or all perfect. Keesha is a person and she is learning and growing and changing. So am I. We have left what I thought of as 'normal' but it is really okay, just as it is."

Example from your life:
Example you've observed in your child or other family member:

What could be done to change it:

3. **Overgeneralization**: Overgeneralizing occurs when we come to a general conclusion based on a single event. Almost any thought can become overgeneralized, and these can be spotted because they tend to include some element of "always" or "never": "It's important to never let anyone down"; "Taking risks is always good/bad." Our brains are hardwired to make generalizations as they help to streamline the effort we put into thinking. There are times when generalizations can help us (e.g., planning for a typical work day), but there are times when overgeneralizing thoughts prevents us from seeing the whole picture. This means that we may not be able to come up with alternative ways of looking at a situation. The tendency to

overgeneralize can lead someone to believe a single, unpleasant incident is part of a never-ending pattern of defeat.

Example: Tasha's use of self-injury to cope with negative feelings led her father, Dwight, to assume that she would always turn to bad habits to cope (he would often think, "she's just a negative person, she will always use negative ways of dealing with life"). He thus had a tendency to assume that any behavior he noticed in Tasha was likely to be somewhat dysfunctional and part of a global pattern of negative coping. This led him to discount or not recognize at all her more constructive habits. This simplistic picture of her abilities meant that he never acknowledged her more positive coping efforts, which led to her feeling overlooked and discounted. This dynamic frustrated both of them, but Dwight was largely unaware of the role he played in perpetuating the frustration.

What Dwight did: Once he began to see that he played a role in setting Tasha up to fail by overgeneralizing and always assuming that she was using negative coping patterns, Dwight worked to actively observe and amplify even small positive actions Tasha took. He also challenged himself to let go of noticing her more negative strategies (like leaving the dinner table early if she was upset by what someone said). He also made a point of making sure Tasha knew that he was noticing her coping strengths by periodically complimenting her on these. It improved their interactions considerably. He had not realized how much his approval mattered to her. It was nice to see her smile once in a while.

Example from your life:
Example you've observed in your child or other family member:

What could be done to change it:

4. **Jumping to conclusions**: This is a close cousin to overgeneralization and occurs when we use limited or even no evidence to support an opinion or to decide how someone else is feeling, what they are thinking, or how they are behaving. These are most commonly negative conclusions. Common examples of jumping to conclusions include assuming that you know what someone else is thinking (often negative) and then basing your reactions on those false conclusions (e.g., "Janie is angry; I am sure it must mean that she does not like me. Why do I always lose friends I like?!").

   Example: Xi was quick to assume that her daughter, Sao, cut when she was angry with Xi for something, even if there was no evidence of this. It made Xi feel like she was walking on eggshells around her daughter all of the time, and this led her to resent Sao.

   What Xi did: Once the family therapist pointed this out in a way Xi could hear it, Xi worked hard to stop making the assumption that every time Sao cut it was because she was upset with her mother. Instead, she worked on checking out her assumption with Sao. She started by being honest with Sao about this automatic assumption and how it made her feel resentful. Sao agreed that she would be honest with her mom when Xi felt a need to check out her fear. It was not always comfortable, but they both found that this simple act of checking out the assumption reduced Xi's fear and resentment and sometimes helped Sao not cut even when she wanted to—just telling her mom that she was feeling the urge helped to decrease it.

Example from your life:
Example you've observed in your child or other family member:

What could be done to change it:

5. **Catastrophizing**: This is best described as expecting disaster to strike, no matter what the evidence says. This often means the thinker magnifies the negative and engages in a lot of future-focused "what-if" scenarios (e.g., "I just know the worst is going to happen! What if people find out and blame me?" "What if it all gets out of control?"). It may also require the thinker to minimize evidence that may run counter to the catastrophic prediction or worry (e.g., "We had a positive conversation yesterday but that really doesn't mean anything"). Needless to say, this can lead to tremendous anxiety.

Example: Maria was certain that her daughter's self-injury meant that she would eventually try to end her life. No matter how Lucia seemed to improve, Maria was convinced that Lucia was getting worse. Lucia felt demoralized, and Maria was hypervigilant and scared.

What Maria did: Once Maria decided to actively work on this, she found it most helpful to be honest about her tendency to assume the worst. Because it was a very strong tendency occurring in multiple areas of her life related to her daughter, she decided to start a journal in which she would write down all of her worst fears. She then worked on separating what she knew was currently happening from something that was not happening and may or may not happen in the future. (For example, her daughter was not currently suicidal. While she had been suicidal more than a year ago while having a hard time with a romantic partner, there was no sign that the suicidal thoughts had come back or would come back soon.)

Maria did this every time she starting to feel a sense of panic or dread about the future. Often just writing it down helped. Sometimes, she needed to check out fears with her daughter or other family members. She slowly began to feel calmer and less worried that something horrible would inevitably happen.

Example from your life:
Example you've observed in your child or other family member:

What could be done to change it:

6. **Personalizing**: Personalizing occurs when one interprets the comments or actions of others as relating to oneself in some way. We may believe that there is a message, usually a slight of some sort, embedded in things people around us say or do. Personalization can also lead us to see ourselves as the cause of external events (e.g., "my child started to self-injure because her dad and I used to fight where she could hear us when she was young"). The tendency to see oneself as the focus or cause of other people's comments or actions can also lead to an unhealthy amount of worry about one's image, especially as it is reflected in one's child.

   Example: Sammy, Darren's daughter, was very direct in her comments and observations, many of which were delivered seemingly without a lot of thought for other people's feelings. Most people who knew her simply thought of it as "just Sammy." Darren, however, had a hard time not taking Sammy's comments personally. Not only did he worry that Sammy's style reflected a failure of his as a parent, but he often assumed that her remarks were intended as a commentary on what he perceived as his failures. For example, when she observed that there was rarely enough good food in the house, he assumed she was criticizing his ability to take care of her. He often felt like she meant to wound him. This made him really reactive and jumpy around her.

What Darren did: Darren began to see that his assumption that Sammy's negative comments were a reflection on or about him was hurting them both. He knew he couldn't change his daughter, and he came to recognize that he could not take what she said so personally. Once he started to explore his reactions, he realized that one of his siblings had a similar style and that Darren had often felt singled out. This was part of the reason he reacted so strongly. That realization made it easier for him to separate Sammy's way of being in the world from anything he had done. He did try to listen to her when she spoke to him directly about something he had done, and it slowly became easier not to take it so personally.

Example from your life:
Example you've observed in your child or other family member:

What could be done to change it:

7. **Blaming**: We hold other people responsible for problems and overlook how we may have contributed to the situation. Or, taking the other tack, we blame ourselves for every problem. This blame game can lead to heavy emotional burdens and feelings of tremendous guilt and anger.

Example: Lucia's perception that Jamal's self-injury was done as a way to hurt her (she personalized it) left her depressed and also resulted in a series of complaints about him to close family members and friends, most often comments about how Jamal "makes her feel bad about herself." Lucia blamed Jamal for a lot of her negative thoughts and feelings and believed life would be much better if Jamal was different. She failed to understand that nobody can "make" us feel any particular way—only we have control over our own emotions and emotional reactions.

What Lucia did: Lucia was often angry with her son, and she knew something had to change. She began to understand and accept that her tendency to blame her son was an example of defensiveness, which had started long before he was born. Working on these patterns while Jamal was in therapy working on his helped her to feel less angry and, eventually, more compassionate for them both.

Example from your life:
Example you've observed in your child or other family member:

What could be done to change it:

8. **"Shoulds" and "musts"**: This is when we have a list of iron-clad rules about how we and others "should" and "must" behave. People who break the rules make us angry, and we feel guilty when we violate these rules ourselves. People may believe they are motivating themselves or others with shoulds and shouldn'ts, but this behavior is rarely motivating and instead

tends to punish before we even get started. For example, "I really should exercise. I shouldn't be so lazy." *Musts* and *oughts* are also offenders. These "rules" often lead to feelings of guilt, anger, frustration, and resentment.

Example: Bonnie felt guilty about her daughter Lynn's mental health challenges. She blamed herself for the difficulties her child had lived through and spent a lot of time trying to make it up to her. When she was honest with herself, she knew that the long list of "should haves" she carried around was weighing her down: "I should have spent more time with her as a child"; "I shouldn't have gone back to work so soon after she was hospitalized"; "A good mom must always be there for her and know what she needs, even if she doesn't know how to ask me for it." Blaming herself was leading Bonnie to resent her daughter, but she did not know how to stop herself from thinking this way and free herself from this negative pattern.

What Bonnie did: Unlike Lucia in the preceding example, Bonnie blamed herself for her child's limitations and vulnerabilities. When she realized that she was holding herself to an unreasonably high standard, she made regular efforts to catch her automatic and often not even fully conscious thoughts and associated emotions. She acknowledged that she had a fairly long list of musts and shoulds for herself and others as well and that this was a source of tension in her relationships. She asked her family and close friends to help her see when she was doing this and vowed to openly listen to their descriptions of her in her "should and must" moments. Over time, she got better at seeing when her musts and shoulds showed up and was able to become more flexible.

Example from your life:
Example you've observed in your child or other family member:

What could be done to change it:

9. **Fallacy of Change**: In this case, we have conscious or unconscious expectations that other people will change in a way that lines up better with our own sensibilities or expectations. We may use various forms of pressure to subtly or not so subtly direct their behavior. In these cases, being "right" is more important than understanding the feelings of others, even loved ones. We may believe that we need them to change in order for us to be content.

Example: Kara always struggled with her son's willfulness. He frequently behaved in ways she very much disliked. When he started self-injuring, she felt both fear and anger. The anger was particularly strong when she felt like she knew exactly what her son needed to do to change. His refusal to do what seemed so clear to her was maddening at times, especially when she was certain that what she had in mind would work for him. This led to feelings of anger at him, too often resulting in fights, but she was not sure how to stop it.

What Kara did: Kara used an approach similar to Bonnie's. When she started to understand that she was very rigid about what she thought was right and wrong, what should and shouldn't be done, and what needed to happen to make something better, Kara asked for her family's and friends' support in helping see when she was in her right/wrong mindset so she could refrain from acting out at her son in those times. It was not always easy to hear her son angrily tell her that she was being rigid, but she worked hard to just stay quiet and listen as much as she could to what he was saying. She also stopped trying to control everything and noticed that other people's ideas often worked out as well if not better than her own. Once her son realized that she would actually listen to him, he started sharing other things as well.

Example from your life:
Example you've observed in your child or other family member:

What could be done to change it:

10. **Emotional Reasoning**: Emotional reasoning involves concluding that one's feelings about something make it true. For instance, having a fearful feeling about something leads to the conclusion that it is dangerous or threatening. Or, having a sense that one's child is a little less talkative at breakfast than usual leads to the conclusion that something bad must have happened the day before. In essence, having an emotion leads to conclusions that may or may not be true but which are assumed to be true because they are felt strongly.

Example: Erika was nervous about her daughter Molly starting at a new school, believing that the stress might trigger a self-injury episode. These insecurities and fears led Erika to assume that Molly was having a hard time at school and resulted in her constantly texting Molly while she was at school to see how she was doing. Molly liked her new school, but her mother's constant texts left Molly worried: "If my mom is this stressed and worried that I can't make it, then I probably won't be able to handle it." Her worry about her mother's worry reinforced her urge to self-injure, and she had to work even harder to resist it.

What Molly did: Once Ericka began to see how her fears were causing her to use faulty reasoning and ultimately feeding into her daughter's fears, Ericka decided to work on recognizing when she was making emotion-based assumptions, checking out her assumptions when she could. For example, instead of assuming that the knot of worry she had in her belly meant that Molly was not adjusting to school well and thus was likely to be injuring, she asked Molly about her experience at school and about her urges to cut. When Molly reassured her that she wasn't having a difficult time, Ericka worked hard to believe it, and, even if she could not totally dispel the worry, she was able to stop constantly checking in on Molly. This helped Molly feel safer and more confident as well as less worried about her mom's own worries.

Example from your life:

Example you've observed in your child or other family member:

What could be done to change it:

A few important and useful themes run through these preceding stories; they can provide insight into how to reduce cognitive distortions that might be making it more difficult for you to support your child. Here are the themes we noted:

Each parent:

- *Had a strong desire to do something differently* and came up with ideas, either alone or in conjunction with someone like a therapist, for addressing the problem in a productive way;
- Realized that positive transformation required *awareness* that their automatic thoughts and emotions were contributing in some way to their child's challenges;
- Exhibited an ability to *understand how their patterns worked* and had to *leverage their strengths* to make positive desired change;
- Had to work on *changing negative thought patterns into more neutral or positive thought patterns;*
- Had to *separate their own experience from their child's;*
- Had to find ways to *recognize progress in themselves* in order to stay engaged with the process, because change is hard;
- Had to *adopt a higher degree of compassion* for themselves and for their children at some point in this process. It really doesn't work very well otherwise.

Some parents strategically used tools, like a journal or regular feedback from family or friends, to support their desired shift. Although this is not always evident at first, many of the parents noticed positive changes in their children and/or their families in response to the changes they were making. This is great reinforcement when it happens!

It is important to note that eliminating all negative thinking is not the primary goal here. Instead, the hope is that you will become more aware of your own patterns of thinking and understand the extent to which they affect your interactions with others, particularly your self-injurious child. Understanding your own tendencies and spotting them in progress will help you control how much power to give them. Likewise, it is important to note that sometimes our more negative thought patterns can provide some meaningful information about us and/or our children (or other loved ones). In these cases, the easiest way to let go of these damaging negative thought patterns is to observe and acknowledge negative perceptions and associated feelings, recognize how these might work to influence your reactions to parenting situations, and to begin to react in more measured, more mindful ways.

With awareness of our own cognitive, emotional, and behavioral limits comes the ability to make more conscious or intentional changes or behaviors. Let's look at an example. One of the most common reactions that parents have when finding out that their child self-injures is anger. For many parents, this reaction is automatic, a gut reaction. Two of our interviewees described their parents' immediate reactions to their self-injury as follows:

> When they first found out, my parents kept on pushing the topic. They said, "We aren't going to leave until you show us your arms." So I showed it to them and my mom immediately started crying, and my dad was like "why the hell are you doing this?" So the way they brought it up wasn't I think the best way. It's embarrassing to show your parents that you are hurting yourself.
>
> —*Veena, age 17*

> My dad judged it and said this is something that young people did and this is stupid and you should be more mature.
>
> —*Jenny, age 16*

While not all parents react like this, and many families recover from such rocky starts, automatic and largely unexamined and unintended reactions to a child's already out of balance behaviors tend to only make the situation worse. For example, Jenny later commented that, in response to her dad's reaction, she felt shut down by her father:

> I felt awful. I felt that I had tried to reach out. I had tried to be brave. I had tried to open a door, and that it had been slammed in my face, and in a way my greatest fears were true. That there was no help to be found in my parents.
>
> —*Jenny, age 16*

Jenny's reaction is common, and beginnings such as this can take a lot of time and effort to correct. Since your child's self-injury is a clear marker that she or he is struggling with emotion regulation, the responsibility lies with you as the parent to step up your abilities in this area. You and your child (and everyone else around you both) will benefit, and your progress in this area also provides a powerful example to your child of how to begin the process of living a more emotionally balanced life.

Identifying Cognitive Distortions and Replacing Automatic Thoughts

Learning how to recognize and work with deep-rooted thought patterns takes both patience and practice. It is an important step in the process of becoming more mindful. To assist you in this, we have designed an activity that builds on the Automatic Thoughts Record presented in Chapter 6. This Automatic Thoughts Record-Expanded (ATR-E), which is located at the end of this chapter, includes a few important additions. First, this worksheet is meant to help you with working on *yourself* rather than focusing solely on helping your child (remember our mantra, "put your own oxygen mask on first"). Second, we've added three important columns. One column is for you to identify the cognitive distortion that is reflected in the thoughts you're having. We find that identifying the cognitive distortion(s) behind the negative thoughts can often help us come up with alternative ways of looking at things. With these replacement thoughts, you're less likely to find yourself experiencing such strong emotions in a given situation, and you will be less likely to overreact during these times. A second column prompts you to consider an alternative way of viewing the situation, and a final column helps you reevaluate your emotional experience once you've considered or tried out these replacement thoughts.

Recognizing and Challenging Core Beliefs

Reviewing information you record on the ATR-E about the cognitive distortions and negative automatic thoughts you experience may make you want to explore how these work in more detail. What patterns do you notice? As you begin to recognize your automatic thoughts, you'll likely also begin to notice patterns. Perhaps, for example, you noticed that many of your cognitive distortions involve feelings of defectiveness, incompetence, or being "less than" (e.g., "I can't get anything right"). A core belief that you are somehow not good enough might be at the root of that cognitive distortion.

Core beliefs are a significant part of who we are. They can arise from experiences we have in childhood, biological predispositions, and cultural influences. Core beliefs can be very positive ("I am lovable," "I am smart") or rather negative ("there is something wrong with me"). While it is beyond the scope of this book to help you with uncovering *why* you may hold particular core beliefs and insecurities, we can point you in the direction of some good resources. Here, we encourage you to use the patterns you may have seen in reflecting on and recording your negative, automatic thoughts to uncover your core beliefs.

> Parents' core beliefs about themselves and their own lives, even aspects of life that seem to have nothing to do with parenting or having children, strongly influence how they parent and what they communicate to their children about life.

For many of us, core beliefs are deeply held and unquestioned; as such they are also often entirely unconscious. They are not, however, passive and inactive. Instead, just as a child's core beliefs are likely to be at the heart of her self-injury story, parents' core beliefs about themselves and their own lives, even aspects of life that seem to have nothing to do with parenting or having children, strongly influence how they parent and what they communicate to their children about life. Indeed, a number of seemingly disparate thoughts can actually be expressions of a core belief that may be entirely unconscious. For example, a parent who unconsciously fears failing in his own life may project that fear onto a child and thus worry in obvious ways about his child's failures. This parent may experience a range of random weekly or even daily worries (e.g., "I would like to apply for that job, but I know I will never be hired," "I better hurry, my partner will be angry if I am late," "I know my boss is mad at me for not getting a report in on time, even though he has not said so") that are all expressions of that single core belief ("I am a failure").

Of course, there always may be reasons for worry, but when thinking patterns become evident, particularly if those worries are ungrounded by any sort of evidence, there is likely a core belief at work. This is one of the reasons why parents' mental health challenges, such as depression (which tends to go along with a lot of negative core beliefs) can make children more vulnerable to depression themselves. Parents, after all, pass along more than their genetic predisposition for physiological traits or disease risk; they also pass along narratives and core beliefs.

Commonly Held Core Beliefs

Core beliefs are often strongly shaped by cultural and family history, and though each individual's beliefs differ, there is a set of core beliefs that are generally common in Western cultures[3] (all cultures have deeply embedded and widely agreed upon cultural narratives and beliefs); these are listed here. Do any of these resonate with you? In addition to simply asking yourself this question as you peruse the list, you can use patterns that emerge from your ATR-E after you have recorded your thoughts for 7–10 days. By looking objectively for patterns in the types of thinking distortions (and negative feelings) you experience, you may find clues about some of your core beliefs. These are examples of relatively common core beliefs that people in Western cultures hold:

Defectiveness. This is the general sense that one is inherently flawed, incapable, or unworthy. Examples of thoughts characteristic to this core belief include, "I'm insignificant"; "I don't deserve anything good"; "I'm useless."

Abandonment. Core beliefs rooted in abandonment assume that people will ultimately leave, which will lead to misery and loneliness. People with abandonment beliefs often feel they are unlovable. They may seek continual reassurance from others and may avoid being honest to prevent being abandoned. Examples of thoughts characteristic to this core belief are: "Anyone who loves me will leave me"; "If I stand up for myself, my partner will leave"; "I can't be happy on my own"; "I'm not as good as other people."

Helplessness/Powerlessness. This core belief is rooted in the assumption that one lacks control and self-efficacy. These beliefs of helplessness often lead to difficulties with transitions and change and can cause some to try to either overcontrol their environments or completely give up. Common thoughts that are characteristic to this core belief are: "I can do nothing to improve my situation"; "I'm trapped and can't find a way out"; "I have no control over my emotions"; "I can't say 'no.'"

Caretaking and/or Self-sacrifice. Caretaking beliefs often show up as taking pride in one's ability to be diligent and dependable and feeling a need to care for others or engage in self-sacrifice. Self-sacrifice beliefs involve an excessive need to forfeit one's own needs. This comes from the belief that we are responsible for the happiness of others. Common thoughts characteristic of this core belief are: "If I don't do it, no one will"; "If I care enough, I can fix it/her/him"; "My needs are unimportant."

Since core beliefs can feel like unmodifiable "truths," it can be helpful to scrutinize and challenge those core beliefs that are potentially compromising your ability to be the parent you want to be. While it may be helpful to consider where core beliefs come from, you need not thoroughly analyze yourself to improve your situation. Change is possible regardless of why you hold these beliefs. Growing awareness of your particular negative thoughts and the underlying core beliefs that may be driving them can be an enriching,

> The slowing down of our automatic thoughts, feelings, and reactions is central to becoming a mindful parent.

lifelong experience. Of course, this type of self-reflection can also be good training to help you discuss with your teen her own thoughts and feelings.

Building a New Way of Seeing

Even small changes and insights can be helpful since they may enable you to pause, take an extra breath, and consider a better course of action in situations in which you might be prone to reacting automatically. Being mindful of these negative, automatic thoughts is the first step toward changing them. As one father reflects on his experiences with his child:

> My child's issues are hers. They affect me. Allowing her to own her issues and working on my issues that became apparent through [therapy] was effective. I made major decisions that changed our living circumstances and helped her understand how important she is. I respect her, and, to my best ability, allow her to be who she is without judgment.
> —*Anil, on learning to maintain healthy boundaries with his child*

Learning how to observe, reflect, and then decide how to best engage is a practice that can be applied to almost any situation, particularly in those that are emotionally challenging. At first this may feel unnatural. When our emotions are strongly activated, it can feel most "right" to *act* in some way—to leave, yell, fight, criticize, or push away. While these are all natural and fairly universal reactions to stress, particularly family-related stress, they are often not helpful. The slowing down of our automatic thoughts, feelings, and reactions is central to becoming a mindful parent, the topic to which we will dedicate the next chapter.

Activities

Activity 1: Automatic Thoughts Worksheet

Take a look at the partially completed Automatic Thoughts Record-Expanded version that follows. Do any of these thoughts look familiar to you? These come from the common experiences of parents relating to their child's self-injury episodes. What thoughts and emotions have you experienced? Now is a good time to reflect and consider the thoughts as they come up, and the feelings you have as a result. Not sure where to start? Think about the last time you experienced a strong negative emotion, such as anger, anxiety, or frustration. What was the situation that led up to your emotions? Can you identify any thoughts you had that may have contributed? Reviewing the list of cognitive distortions we provided earlier in this chapter may also help you to pinpoint some of the thoughts that you may have had at the time. Once you've identified the type of cognitive distortion that may have been driving your thoughts, then it becomes easier to consider a replacement thought. We have also included a blank record to record your own ATR-E (you can make multiple copies to use as independent worksheets).

Automatic Thoughts Record—Expanded						
Date/Time	Situation	Automatic Thought	Emotion(s)	Cognitive Distortion	Replacement Thoughts	Emotion(s)
	What led to the change in your mood? What distressing physical sensations did you experience?	What thoughts or images went through your mind? On a scale from 0–100, how much did you believe them at the time?	What emotions did you feel at the time? On a scale from 0–100, how intense were the emotion(s)?	What cognitive distortion(s) can you identify in your thoughts?	What alternative thoughts can you identify that might help to explain your perceptions of the situation?	What emotions do you feel now? From 0–100, how intense are these emotions?
Friday, 11/4 5 pm	Noticed new cuts on my child's wrist	"She's never going to get better; she's out of control" "I am heartbroken" "What is wrong with our family?!"80	Anxiety, guilt, fear, anger 100	Labeling, overgeneralization	"She has made progress over the past couple of months. She is really trying, but is having a difficult time right now. This is a bump in the road and she and I are both learning skills along the way to help ourselves"	Compassion 50
Tuesday 11/8, 3:30 pm	My child threatened to cut again if I did not do what he wanted	"He is manipulating me"70	Anger, anxiety	Personalization	"His behavior is a sign that he is feeling overwhelmed. I can be steady and strong to allow him to sort through this"	Calm, occasionally nervous 60

Automatic Thoughts Record—Expanded

Date/Time	Situation	Automatic Thought	Emotion(s)	Cognitive Distortion	Replacement Thoughts	Emotion(s)
	What led to the change in your mood? What distressing physical sensations did you experience?	What thoughts or images went through your mind? On a scale from 0–100, how much did you believe them at the time?	What emotions did you feel at the time? On a scale from 0–100, how intense were the emotion(s)?	What cognitive distortion(s) can you identify in your thoughts?	What alternative thoughts can you identify that might help to explain your perceptions of the situation?	What emotions do you feel now? From 0–100, how intense are these emotions?

Again we'll stress that attending to your internal dialogue and negative automatic thoughts is a skill that takes time and practice. By using the ATR-E on a daily basis, noticing your thoughts will get easier. For many parents, this may be enough to focus on. Simply recording thoughts and looking for negative, automatic thinking patterns will help you in your interactions with others and in managing your emotions and mood. It is important to note that when you rate your emotional experience after doing this exercise, you should find that your 0–100 emotion rating is *lower* than it was when you first rated your emotions. If it's not, then you will want to consider coming up with other replacement thoughts that allow you a different perspective and alleviate negative emotions (and, subsequently, that emotion rating). Understanding your negative thought patterns will help you help your child with his or hers.

10

Becoming a Mindful Parent

Strategies and Skills for Parenting a Child Who Self-Injures

When we practice mindfulness, we learn that much of the chatter of the mind is just that: chatter. It's not reality—it's worry, it's anxiety, it's baseless projection. Mindfulness teaches <people> to be aware of their thoughts, perhaps simply labeling them as "worrying." They can acknowledge anxiety, without getting caught up in the negative thoughts it generates.

—Sarah Rudell Beach, creator of LeftBrainBuddha.com

Growing Mindful Parenting Skills

This chapter is dedicated to building your own mindfulness skills and to introducing the idea of "mindful parenting." We provide strategies and tools throughout that can help you to become more mindful and to deepen your mindful parenting skills. First, we introduce you to various ways that you can build mindfulness into your daily routine (don't worry, we know that your time is a precious and limited commodity, so we're realistic about how to fit practice into a busy schedule). Second, we spend time working on the important skill of *listening* to family members and *hearing* not just the words they are saying, but what intentions and feelings are behind them. Finally, we return to the thoughts, feelings, and actions that you have identified as difficult in earlier worksheets. Based on these, we aim to help you to develop intention-setting skills for helping to resolve difficulties and achieve goals.

What Is Mindfulness?

The practice of mindfulness is defined by psychologist Jon Kabat-Zinn as "the awareness that emerges through paying attention, on purpose, in the present moment, and nonjudgmentally to the unfolding of experience moment by moment."[1] The idea is that "being mindful" will lead to greater awareness of thoughts, feelings, and sensations and that, this, in turn, will reduce anxiety and enhance a sense of well-being. Mindfulness skills are widely recognized to be developed and refined through *intentional* deployment of attention—the act of strengthening control over the wanderings and activities of one's mind; it is the practice of giving full and exclusive attention to *what is happening right now.* Mindfulness techniques are at the heart of at least some of the therapeutic techniques your child will encounter in therapy. For instance, as discussed in Chapter 7, the most common approach to treating self-injury is known as dialectical behavioral therapy (DBT for short), which includes mindfulness as a core component.

> Mindfulness techniques can be very useful when dealing with stressful situations and are likely to be helpful in leading to more productive communications with your child.

Mindfulness techniques can be very useful when dealing with stressful situations and are likely to be helpful in leading to more productive communications with your child because they promote more flexible thinking; this increased flexibility comes in very handy when parenting self-injurious youth. More flexible thinking can lead to:

- Greater acceptance of situations you cannot control.
- Enhanced ability to smoothly transition from one situation or scene to another.
- Reduced likelihood of overreacting to our own feelings and thoughts (the internal landscape) and to what happens in the world around us (the external landscape).

Practicing mindfulness is associated with greater levels of positive mood, lower levels of anxiety and depression, and greater satisfaction with relationships as well as decreases in physiological markers of stress and more activity in the parts of the brain responsible for self-awareness, compassion, planning, judgment, emotion regulation, learning, and memory.[2] Moreover, it does not require a lot of effort to learn. Indeed, recent research indicates that as little as 12 minutes of meditation a day over an 8-week period may be enough to create changes in the brain's gray matter, leading to improvements in memory, sense of self, and empathy. One of the most prominent results of regularly practicing mindfulness is that it becomes easier to observe what is happening objectively, in oneself and in relationships, and mindfulness practice makes it easier to respond with kindness, empathy, equanimity, and patience. This feature of mindfulness is immensely helpful in emotionally charged family situations. Learning to detach from the emotional pull of a situation while also experiencing a sense of compassion will heighten your ability to understand and respond to yourself and your own family in a thoughtful, grounded way— regardless of the frustration and conflict you may have all experienced in the past.

While a broad review of mindfulness is more than we can do here, we want to introduce one of the mindfulness-based models used in DBT[3] called "observe, describe, engage" (or OBE for short). We like this because it is fairly easy to remember and it is a really useful parenting guide in stressful moments. Here are the steps:

- *Observe*: Slow down, observe without doing.
- *Describe*: Detach from an immediate highly emotional outcome and take the time you need to calmly assess the best course of action.
- *Engage*: Show patience, kindness, and persistence to both yourself and your child.

Used consistently, this technique is a great way to navigate charged situations in a nonjudgmental way that builds communication and empathy and strengthens the parent–child relationship. Of course, while many of these skills can be practiced and developed in collaboration with your child, you may find that even if you don't have her cooperation and involvement, the benefits to you and your relationships with others will be evident. Using this approach will also benefit your child—who is learning by watching you—in developing skills for dealing with stress, conflict, and intense negative feelings.

What Is the Link Between Mindfulness and Parenting?

Much of the traditional behavior modification and parenting literature emphasizes the use of reinforcement (such as praise, incentives, rewards) to increase desirable behaviors and punishment or consequences (such as time out, loss of privileges) to decrease undesirable behaviors. But while these strategies can work well for younger children, they often leave parents of teens and young adults struggling with how to address their child's behavior in a more nuanced manner and how to better connect with and relate to their kids.

The key to parenting mindfully is being able to listen to your children, understand the underlying emotions involved, and accept everything with as much compassion and equanimity as you can. Since you are also present, it is important to include and accept your own feelings and perspectives as well.[4]

Consistent use of mindfulness practices will help cultivate awareness of multiple perspectives and settle into a more peaceful, steady state of mind that tends to reduce stress and increase honest communication with your child and others. The goal of mindfulness is not to change your real feelings or abilities, but instead to authentically acknowledge and accept them. These insights can lead to significant positive changes in a variety of areas.

> The goal of mindfulness is not to change your real feelings or abilities but to authentically acknowledge and accept them.

Learning how to become mindful can take practice. It is not, however, difficult—at least not in a way that most of us are accustomed to. For example, one might decide to work toward reducing time spent ruminating—broadly defined as revisiting stressful thoughts over and over. This means learning to be conscious of where one directs one's attention (e.g., away from rumination and negative thoughts and toward thoughts and actions that support more positive feelings and behaviors; this is real work for most of us!). It also means supporting this effort with purposeful practices, such as making regular time for meditation or other physical activities (such as a 30-minute walk) that quiet our stressful thoughts.

How Do I Become More Mindful?

There are a growing number of mindfulness approaches. Rather than review them all here, we will share three foundational skills common across most of them. Our goal is not to teach a mini-mindfulness course, but to help you understand the basic principles for yourself and in relation to your parenting goals. We also provide at the end of the chapter a few easy activities you might use to become acquainted with each skill.

Cultivate Present Moment Awareness: Learn to Become the Observer

Present moment awareness is primarily about *observing*. It requires directing one's full attention to sensations happening right here and right now (sounds, smells, visuals, touch, taste). Or it may involve "observing" your own thoughts or feelings as they occur in real time. It is the opposite of multitasking. While it is easiest to begin with observing what our senses are telling us, we must also develop the ability to *observe our thoughts but not react to them*. The trick for most of us is learning how to *watch only*, keeping the mind from making judgments about what it is observing. The mind can watch but not evaluate or criticize. This is much harder to do than it seems!

Build an Acceptance-Oriented, Nonjudgmental Perspective: Learn to Step Back and Describe

Once present moment awareness becomes more comfortable, it is helpful to work on using that expanded awareness to identify and diffuse automatic negative thoughts and feelings. This often requires accepting what we cannot change about ourselves, our lives, or other people and allowing that surrender to make space for more understanding and compassion—for others and for ourselves. It is amazing what this seemingly small shift can do. Evaluating— judging in negative and positive ways—every observation and experience that we have is so ingrained in us that we are often un- aware we are doing it. And, since negative thoughts and emotions are more "sticky" than positive emotions (meaning we notice and remember them better than we do positive experiences and emotions), they often dominate in the form of judgments, critical analysis, or negative expectations. Mindfulness invites us to work on not evaluating or reacting to what we observe—in ourselves or others—and to replace our judgments with curiosity, compassion, and/or simple acceptance.

Learning how to simply *be* in an experience, even if it is uncomfort- able, without needing to immediately react or judge is a little easier if we allow ourselves to simply *describe* what is happening without evaluating the inherent goodness or badness of the experience (e.g., "I am feeling extremely frustrated right now because this has happened so many times. I feel trapped in this dynamic"). This helps keep the mind busy (since it has a very hard time being quiet anyway!) and can reinforce attention to the present moment. As Marsha Linehan, the creator of DBT, writes in her DBT skills training manual,[5] in- tention requires "entering wholly and with awareness into life itself, nonjudgmentally, in the present moment. It is the ultimate goal of mindfulness." Observing and describing can happen almost simul- taneously, but describing helps to draw our attention away from our feelings and toward the simple act of observing what is occurring inside the body or in the outside world. In this stance, there is a clear, identifiable part of you that is simply watching, as though you are watching a movie.

Set the Stage for Effective Engagement: Learn How to Respond from a Place of Authentic Care

Once we learn to quiet the mind, center it in the present, and simply allow what is present to be there without strong reactions or judgments, it becomes possible for us to respond to situations in less emotionally charged ways. "Engaging" means that you participate by bringing yourself fully into the current moment with as much peace and calm as possible. But this is more than simply demonstrating calmness. It is action with *intent to communicate care, concern, and respect for oneself and others,* even if the conversation is difficult or if the right action is likely to elicit protest or short-term anger (like having to refuse a child some desired object or experience). It is important to know that engaging in this way does not mean you are a pushover or that you are overly "nice" or that you avoid doing or saying things which are likely to be controversial. Indeed, sometimes it requires difficult conversations.

Foundational intention refers to those qualities, characteristics, or experiences we hold closest to our hearts and which transcend particular situations or relationships.

A key element of mindful engagement requires being able to identify and hold awareness of a set of core intentions and values. This can be difficult at first since most of us do not spend much time figuring out what our most foundational intentions and values are. In the broadest and simplest terms, *foundational intention* refers to those qualities, characteristics, or experiences we hold closest to our hearts and which transcend particular situations or relationships. "Foundational" refers to the idea that these are a set of intentions that reflect core life values (e.g., to have loving, mutually respectful relationships) rather than objects of experience or desire (e.g., to become an engineer). We often have intentions for our lives, our children, and our work that we cannot always articulate but which deeply influence our thoughts, feelings, and actions. Many of these are overlapping, but sometimes they are distinct. We are often most aware of these unarticulated intentions when we act in ways that undermine or thwart them. For example, I may place a high value on being a loving parent and may not remember this until I experience remorse for losing my temper and yelling at my child. It is very helpful for parents to identify those values they hold most dear and to hold them in mind when they engage with a child since it can help to keep them calm, centered, and mindful of longer term parenting goals.

Mindfully Parenting a Child who Self-Injures

I listen more. I've learned to shut up and listen to her.
—Mwenda, on learning to listen to her child

And while it's really hard, you really have to try not to act emotionally and even times I've said to Jessica, "Okay, I need to think about this, I can't talk to you about it now, I'll talk to you about it in the morning," to put it off because, I mean, emotionally, you just want to say, "Why are you doing that?!" you know and just exploding is not going to help it. And that's gonna draw them further back, so take a breath and take a minute. You know, I thought I was pretty savvy, and I have two college degrees in communication, and I have been working now almost 34 years with students and kids and families, and it got by me!
—Shelly, on learning to stay present and centered with her child.

So, how do we apply these skills to a parenting context? In many ways, there is no better place to practice these skills than in parenting. That is doubly true when parenting youth who struggle with one or more mental health challenges since being mindful offers many opportunities to practice observing, detaching, describing, and responding from a more centered place. While the mindful parenting activities we have included in this chapter are largely focused on teaching you to apply these skills on your own, you can use the same techniques with your child (or anyone in your life, for that matter). It's also important to understand that the foundation of parenting mindfully is less about specific words or actions and more about a state of mind or mental orientation. The insights and awareness you glean from each of the skill areas will shape the actions and verbal exchanges that happen when you are with your child.

For example, when working on the skill of cultivating present moment awareness, you can practice simply observing (without judging) your child's emotional state or reaction, your child's physical behavior, or anything else going on before you. You can also bring your awareness to your own emotional or physical reaction. You may become aware that you are frustrated and angered by your daughter's words and behaviors, for instance. When engaged in active observing, however, you simply see and note this experience without adding additional thoughts or commentary or outwardly reacting. Observing and not reacting is challenging and something that requires practice. It is preferable to begin using these skills during times of low stress, if possible. Then, as you become more comfortable using the skills and they become more natural for you, it will be easier to use them in more challenging, high stress encounters.

> Observing and not reacting is challenging and something that requires practice.

Once you can simply observe for several moments or more, you can work on describing the situation to yourself in a way that does not stoke strong emotion. The goal here is not to justify your response or talk yourself down, it is simply to extend the observing stance into a nonjudgmental description of what is occurring. For example, a parent whose child is reactive, loud, and angry about something may describe the situation to her- or himself this way: "My child is angry and is yelling at me. I feel my stomach and chest getting tight, and I think my pulse is rising. I feel afraid that she is going to cut again, and I feel like I should stop her from being angry so that she won't do that."

Observing and describing are really helpful in slowing down the reaction process, stepping away from the flurry of emotions that often make a hard situation even harder, and allowing the body and feelings to calm down a little. Simply taking the time to describe the situation to yourself as though you were describing the scene and characters in a movie slows down the emotional reaction and makes it easier for you to stay present in the face of your child's outburst without becoming defensive and embattled in argument.

Maintaining this kind of distance is an essential part of assuming a nonjudgmental and accepting stance. This can be very difficult to do when one is the target of another person's anger or hostility, even if it is unspoken. And expecting to be fully accepting or nonjudgmental may simply not be possible if there is a lot of strong emotional activity (e.g., yelling or blaming) going on. But, with some practice, one can use the observe and describe approach to get through the very hard emotional moments and then ease into whatever level of acceptance and nonjudgment is possible. Here is an example:

> Shawna and Greg had been fighting about their daughter, Jenni, for more than a year. Things were frequently tense between them, particularly when Jenni did something that stirred things up. Shawna and Greg had very different ways of understanding and dealing with Jenni, and they simply could not come to agreement about how to present a united front for their daughter.
>
> In a particularly difficult exchange, Shawna felt herself ready to lose it with Greg. She really did not want to replay their drama, so instead of venting her frustration through her words or actions, she took a minute to describe to herself the scene, "Greg is across the room by the mirror. His voice and the look on his face convey his anger and frustration. It is a beautiful day outside but all I see is his anger and all I feel is my own. I cannot see my face, but I am sure that anyone looking at me would see my frustration and anger as well." Taking a minute to describe the scene drew Shawna's thoughts away from the source of her frustration and helped her distance herself from the intensity of her anger. She then told Greg that she needed a little time, left the room, and went outside to breathe. While she was there she observed and described to herself what she saw and felt: birds in the trees, a gentle wind, a slight chill to the air. When her mind came back to the situation with Greg and Jenni, she was more relaxed and had achieved a less reactive distance from the intensity of the feelings.

Since resistance and judgment change almost nothing and often exacerbate tensions, they tend to serve only our short-term need to express frustration. While understandable, it is worthwhile to learn how to quickly recognize what needs to be accepted and what can be productively discussed. Over time, it becomes easier to achieve a sense of inner acceptance and peace *before* action of any sort occurs.

This can be immensely helpful. Taking this time for yourself to clear your head and heart before coming back around to your child or other loved one is always time well spent.

Once you are as centered as you can be and feel ready to respond in a balanced way, you can work on engaging with your child (or others) from a place of authentic care. Within the parenting context, this is most possible when you can keep your loftiest and long-term parenting goals in mind (e.g., "I want my daughter to be emotionally stable and to be healthfully self-sufficient" or "I want my son to be respectful of others"). It sounds easy, but it can be challenging. Take, for example, a situation where a parent worries that imposing consequences for breaking a family agreement or rule will cause his or her child to cut or act out in another way. This often leads to either inaction or angry action since a parent can feel trapped or wedged between two bad options. This happened with Tim when his daughter Lane snuck out of the house to be with a friend late at night. Tim was really angry but also very hesitant to impose a consequence for fear that Lane would start cutting again. When practicing mindful parenting, a parent in this situation would likely acknowledge the fear (that the child may self-injure), accept this as a possibility, and do what she or he ultimately felt was the most right, which very well may mean risking more self-injury. In Tim's case, he decided that there had to be a consequence for breaking a family agreement or rule. Since he was really focused on helping Lane to feel loved and connected to the family, he looked for consequences that may enhance Lane's sense of connection. So, in addition to losing her cell phone for a few days, Tim required Lane to spend time working in the garden with him over the weekend and required her to go grocery shopping with her grandmother. He also allowed her to earn her cell phone back a little earlier by having an honest conversation with him about what was happening for her emotionally and socially, areas she was typically very private about.

Finding ways to leverage whatever influence you may have can be extremely beneficial all around. In addition, you are working to create a fair and consistent environment for your child by setting the tone for healthy communications and expression of emotions. Punishing just to punish or only to express

> When you are not sure about how to react from a centered place, it is better to not react at all.

anger is rarely beneficial in advancing our highest desires for our children, ourselves, or our families.

That said, it is helpful to keep in mind that you do not need to *do* anything in tense or highly emotional moments, even if it feels like you do (or if your child demands it). When you are not sure about how to react from a centered place, it is better to not react at all. The more you can slow down and take a step back to simply observe, process, and mindfully decide how to engage in a way that advances your longer term parenting goals, the less reactive and more constructive and honest the whole exchange is likely to be. We cannot emphasize enough how much a simple change in orientation, coupled with some deep breathing when you are feeling charged up, can make a very big difference in relationship quality. The calmness that comes as part of this practice will help to introduce clarity over time. Not only will your actions from a centered, integrity-filled place be different from what they would be if they had been motivated by a reactive or defensive stance, but your very approach actively models to your child a powerful and healthy way to deal with overwhelming emotions and stress.

Let's turn now to several activities you can use to enhance your mindful parenting skills.

Mindful Parenting Activity: Setting Mindful Parenting Intentions

> So I've learned to not completely push it [self-injury] out of my head but to really try to be more present, really listen, and take action quicker when she's saying something that is—I mean even little things like "My eyes hurt. I need different contacts. Can you make the appointment?" Yeah. Instead of waiting a week, you know, I just do it now.
>
> —Shanti, on learning to stay present and centered with her child

Setting explicit parenting intentions will help guide your actions, particularly when deciding on the right course of action may be hard, such as in times of stress or emotional confusion. Most parenting intentions are not concrete goals, per se (e.g., I want my child to get straight A's); rather, they are ideals we try to embody, model, and teach. For example, it is common for parents to say that they want children to be respectful and/or good students and friends. Our intentions are based on our personal values or ideas about what makes a life successful and worth living. Intention setting is different from goal setting, in that intentions allow a mindful, deliberate, and on-going approach to what we hope to achieve and how we want to live. Goal setting, on the other hand, focuses on the end point and often sets us up for failure since success depends on whether we achieved the goal. Intentions are designed with the journey in mind, rather than the destination.

Quick practice exercise: Take a few minutes right now to think about your parenting intentions for this period of your and your child's life. They may not be the same as they were when your child was young or before she started struggling with self-injury, and that is okay. Take a moment to answer these four reflection questions:

- What core life principles and values do you want to teach your child? Write down three to five examples.

- Which two of these are most important to you in this period of your and your child's life?

- Take a minute to think about how you model these two principles in your daily life with your child (e.g., if you value respect, how do you demonstrate respect to them?). Write down your thoughts on this.

• Think about what you do that may not be totally in alignment with your core parenting intentions. Write down 1–2 examples here for your own reflection.

As you consider your intentions for parenting, use this time to consider the bigger picture of your life and your family's life together. Setting your intentions will help you with establishing a general course of action that you propose to follow. This allows some flexibility within daily schedules and busy lives and an element of forgiveness for things we may not do as perfectly or as well as we would like.

Mindful Parenting Activity: Communicating

> *We are finding better and more ways to communicate. And we are listening more. I ask my daughter often, "Where are you right now?" "How are you really doing?" I call it my pulse check with her. I am not afraid to ask direct questions. We can talk about anything.*
> —Bruno, on family communications

Once you are clear about your foundational intentions and values, it is helpful to be able to communicate them clearly. Mindful parenting is both an inner orientation and a way to approach the outer world. While there are no "do's and don'ts," there are a few communication qualities that increase the likelihood that positive and effective exchange happens. The first step is getting to know your current communication preferences, so, before we delve into the communication techniques that best constitute mindful parenting, let's take a moment to assess what is most comfortable for you now. Becoming aware of your preferred ways to communicate and your strengths and limitations in communicating, both overtly and more subtly, will ultimately provide you with more options for growth and development in this area.

Quick practice exercise: The list here is meant to help you honestly assess some elements of your style and preferences when interacting with your child and will help you assess your strengths and limitations in mindfully communicating with her. These are meant as a tool, not as a test, so there is no formal scoring guide. The aim is to think about each question and to answer honestly (and mindfully!), allowing you to better understand what is working well—and not so well—in your communications with your child.

Communication Strategies

Review the following and rate each mindful communication strategy, *considering how your child would rate you:*	**0:** I never do this **1:** I do not do this so well **2:** I am okay at this **3:** I am really good at this
1. Do you typically make eye contact when you are speaking with your child?	0 1 2 3
2. Do you use a calm, respectful voice?	0 1 2 3
3. Do you respect your child's behavior, waiting to discuss matters with him or her only when he or she is not in a group?	0 1 2 3
4. Do you take responsibility for your part in the mistakes your child makes?	0 1 2 3
5. Do you try to see your child's point of view?	0 1 2 3
6. Do you work to make sure a message of LOVE comes through in your communications?	0 1 2 3
7. Are you a positive thinker, seeing the many positives that your child does?	0 1 2 3
8. Do you set a good example for your child by "owning" your own problems and asking for help?	0 1 2 3

9. Do you listen to what your child has to say and avoid interrupting?	0 1 2 3
10. Do you find yourself fully listening to your child even though there may be many other demands placed on you?	0 1 2 3
11. Do you offer encouragement and acknowledge their efforts?	0 1 2 3
12. When you are upset with your child, do you notice how you are feeling *before* you take action?	0 1 2 3
13. Are you aware of how your moods affect the way you treat your child?	0 1 2 3
14. When engaged in an activity with your child, do you take your time and show that you are attentive to him or her?	0 1 2 3
15. Before you react in a discussion, do you consider your highest intentions?	0 1 2 3

Notice the items on which you are already strong, those on which you could improve, and those on which you know you do not do so well. Do you see any patterns? We have categorized these items into four important areas of mindful parenting. Consider which of these four areas you are doing well in and which you may want to improve:

- *Awareness & present-centered attention*: Items 1, 10, 13, 14
- *Acceptance*: Items 4, 5, 8, 9
- *Nonreactivity*: Items 2, 3, 6, 12
- *Positive parenting*: Items 7, 11, 15

Can you think about specific examples of each area in your own parenting relationship? Although our tendency is to immediately look for the items on which we scored low, take time to also notice what you identified as your strengths—these are important skills that will come in handy in times of stress; since they may come more easily to you, you can rely on them to help you through challenging times.

If you want to take it one step further, pick a few areas in which you want to grow. Maybe these are those items on which you rated yourself lowest, but you may find that you want to improve or grow even stronger in those "middle of the road" areas as well. No parent is fully mindful all of the time. The goal here is not to be perfectly mindful, but to enhance self-awareness. Once you have identified areas for focus, you can start practicing immediately with your child (or with other people in your life—mindful interactions are universally applicable and beneficial). You can visit this list as many times as you want for new ideas and areas of improvement (and gratitude)!

Mindful Parenting Activity: Acceptance and Nonjudgment Through Deep Listening

The self-injury was terrifying for me initially, but proved to be just the tip of the iceberg of her issues. I have more understanding and compassion for her experience now, her fragility, and have more realistic expectations for what our relationship is or could become. I do not believe we will ever trust each other enough to be close, but I believe we will continue to have contact if and when she moves out.

—Mario, on coming to terms with his daughter's self-injury

Moving from a place of disbelief, resistance, or strong negative emotion into a place of acceptance can be very challenging. This is especially true when it comes to parenting since no one can get under our skin as fast as our family members—for better or for worse! Because of this, acceptance and nonjudgment can be difficult to apply. And this skill area is not easy to master; practice is a must. We can, however, work on a few key components of acceptance and nonjudgment through *deep listening* and mindful communication.

So much of what we say to one another is said "between the lines"—in gestures, facial expressions, pauses, and long sighs. If we are oblivious to these communications, or choose not to listen, we are missing out on opportunities to connect in ways that enhance our relationships. The greatest gifts you can give your teen are your time, your presence, your full undivided attention, and total acceptance of who he is, warts and all.

> Deep listening involves learning to connect with your child, to communicate that you care and that you are present.

Deep listening involves learning to connect with your child, to communicate that you care and that you are present. It is a very active process in which one listens with the sole aim of deeply understanding. It is also an excellent mindfulness activity because it requires full presence and attention and thus communicates loving regard.

How do you do it? The trick to deep listening is to be as present and "empty" of thought or running commentary as possible when hearing what someone else is saying. You should not be planning what to say next or reinterpreting what is being said to reinforce your own theories or assumptions. While the deep listener may be experiencing strong thoughts or emotions, he or she practices letting them go and focusing on trying to understand, from the speaker's perspective, what is being shared and what it means to the speaker. While deep listening sounds reasonably straightforward and easy, it is not. If it feels easy then one is probably not doing it correctly (unless you're already schooled in this process, and even veterans can improve).

Deep listening often brings on surprising but common experiences. For example, you are likely to perceive a much fuller range of communications from the person speaking. You will likely notice his words, of course, but you will also probably notice other, more subtle things as well—tone of voice, hand or eye patterns (such as looking away from your eyes when speaking about a shaming event), or other small bodily movements that communicate something that you may have been missing until now. You may intuit things about other people and/or what they're trying to communicate that you did not expect.

These experiences pave the way for several responses. One may be to listen and use your full attention to simply assure the other person that he is heard. You may choose to reflect back what you have heard by offering your interpretation in a way that shows you deeply listened but that stops short of commentary or opinion: "it sounds like you feel really hurt by what happened." Don't feel like you need to restate or parrot their communications back to them; we've found that it's easy to become wrapped up in focusing only on the words being spoken, meaning your focus is less on underlying intent or other subtle cues, and you're focusing more on how to respond. This is not deep listening.

Open, Honest Questions

You may elect to ask "open honest questions."[6] These are questions asked with no agenda and often come up spontaneously as you are listening. *Open, honest questions are intended to help the person who is speaking more than to satisfy your own curiosity or to convey your opinion.* They help the other person explore his beliefs, convictions, and perceptions and may also generate new insights or reveal inner resources of which the speaker was not aware. Here are a few guidelines for open, honest questioning:

1. The best mark of an open, honest question is that you cannot anticipate the answer, nor do you have an expectation for what the answer should be (e.g., *What was easy? What was difficult? What surprised you? What did you learn?*).
2. Stay with the person's language (e.g., *You said this was an impossible situation. Could you say more about what that means to you?*)
3. Rather than only asking questions related to the problem or issue being raised, ask questions directed to the person as well (e.g., *What in your life brings you joy? What would a really good day look like for you?*)
4. Yes/no or right/wrong questions tend to close down inquiry. Instead, ask questions that help open or expand his thinking about the issue or his options.
5. Offer images or metaphors that might engage the person's imagination (e.g., *If you were writing a book about this experience, what might you title the book? Name this chapter?*)
6. Trust your own intuition. Listen deeply and allow questions to come from your heart, not just your head.

Quick practice exercise : The goal of this activity is simple: to practice listening to someone with full attention and with the intention to deeply understand what is being conveyed through words and in more subtle ways.

Step 1: Identify someone in your life with whom you want to practice. This can be a family member or friend, but should be someone who you genuinely want to listen to (at least at the beginning—practice doing this with someone you are not keen on listening to as you progress).

Step 2: Tell her that you are practicing a deep listening technique and invite her to share something that's on her mind; it may or may not have anything to do with you.

Step 3: While it is okay to ask clarifying questions, try first to listen to what is said. If she pauses, then practice staying quiet to allow for more. Often, pauses are reflection points, and there may be more that comes out afterward. If you are not clear about whether you have reached the natural endpoint, feel free to ask something like, "Have you shared everything you are comfortable sharing right now?"

Step 4: Once she is done, you can either thank her for sharing, reflect back what you heard (it is nice in this case to ask if she is okay with that), or ask open, honest questions.

Step 5: If you told her that you were practicing a new communication technique, then you might ask her whether she felt heard by you more than she usually does.

What comes as a result of deep listening is a level of understanding that feels new, fresh, and much more robust than what many of us are accustomed to. The conversation that can occur in the wake of deep listening is often authentic, honest, and usually much more useful and satisfying than what has come to be normal conversation.

For most of us, it takes practice. One knows that it is happening when (a) it feels like work to some degree, (b) one hears "new" information or has a new epiphany or insight, and (c) one feels like he or she is "seeing through another's eyes" for a little while. It is an exceptionally helpful tool to use and often leads to deeper awareness, understanding, and important but previously unasked questions.[6]

Mindful Parenting: Catching the Positives to Improve Your Mood and Parenting Communications

The science of positive thinking indicates that the more we focus our attention on "catching the positives," the more positive emotions we will experience, which in turn broadens our cognitive capacity, stabilizes emotions, and fosters creativity.[7] Remember, words power our thoughts.

If we continually focus on the negatives in our lives, ours and others' shortcomings, and how we don't measure up, then our attention will remain focused on these negative dimensions.

Quick practice exercise: Make a list of the positives you want to catch or grow in your child. Perhaps you're interested in encouraging respectfulness, or responsibility, or kindness? List up to five to focus on catching in your child. Over the next few days, practice being mindful of any and all positive steps your child takes. When you see it, record it in your journal and find a way to communicate to your child that you noticed. No matter what his age, your child will notice and appreciate the positive attention.

Walking the Talk

One of the most powerful means by which we convey intentions and values is through our own behavior. It is a very human thing to say one thing and do another; we all do this. When it comes to parenting, particularly in hard times, it is helpful to work on "walking the talk"—or, in this case, what we hope to help our kids learn about how to live successfully. This is called "social learning"—the idea that people learn through observation (of parents and friends; of TV or the Internet).

Social learning works best when what we do is consistent with what we say. Parents do not have control over all of their children's social interactions, but we have some control over our own attitudes and behaviors. It is important to be conscious of whether we are modeling the behavior and attitudes we hope to teach because this is the very best way for us to reach our parenting goals and to stay connected with the good intentions we have for our children.

Activities

Activity #1: Learn to Become the Observer

You can practice right now by sitting quietly, ideally in a quiet space, for 3–5 minutes (for a real challenge try doing this in a non-quiet place!). Feel free to set an alarm if you have limited time and you don't think the alarm will be a distraction. Ideally, you will sit in an upright position with your head balanced comfortably over your shoulders and your shoulders balanced over your hips, so that you are leaning neither forward nor back. Sitting on a pillow so that your knees are a little lower than your hips and with your back against a wall can provide the support needed to ensure your body is comfortable.

Close your eyes and bring your awareness to your breathing, in and out, for 3–5 minutes. It is natural for your mind to wander—to your to-do lists, recent events, feelings, and the like. Your goal is not to suppress your thoughts but to simply let them come and go without following them. This can be challenging. If you find yourself starting to focus too much on a thought or image, try to bring yourself back. It helps to simply listen to the sound of your breath moving in and out or to focus your attention on the sensations in your feet, then your ankles, then calves, and so on up your body. This way your mind has a task (minds like to be busy!).

When you are done, take another minute or two to review or record what you noticed. This is a very basic practice that helps soothe the central nervous system and cultivates a more mindful perspective. Practicing this way for just 15 minutes a day has been shown to improve cognitive and emotional functioning and interpersonal relationships.

Activity 2: Learn to Step Back and Describe

The goal of this activity is to help you map your thoughts. It will assist you in discovering patterns in where your thoughts are straying (i.e., drifting to the past or future), how much this is happening, and to what extent your stray thoughts are stressful in some form or another (for instance, to-do lists, "shoulds," judgments, or destructive impulses). It ends with an exercise for fostering gratitude for positive, uplifting thoughts and "simple acceptance" of the more stressful thoughts and the feelings they can bring. It requires about 15 minutes of your time. You will need only a pen, paper, and a timer.

1. Begin by spending 3 minutes jotting down a list of all of your thoughts.

2. At the end of 3 minutes, go down your list and label each thought dealing with the *past* with a *"P,"* label thoughts dealing with the *here and now* with an *"N,"* and thoughts of the *future* with an *"F."*

3. Now add up how many of your thoughts fall into each of these categories: P, N, F.

4. How were your thoughts divided? Were most of the thoughts in the past, the now, or the future? Why do you think this is so? There's no use ridiculing yourself for not being able to keep yourself in the present moment. Instead, focus on gently pulling yourself back to the present when you find your thoughts drifting to the past or the future.

5. Now return to your list of thoughts. Review each thought and note with a *"J"* whenever that thought involved a judgment of some sort. Are these judgmental thoughts more likely to occur alongside thoughts about the past, the future, or the present? Why do you think this is so? Judgmental, negative thoughts are more likely to flow from negative ruminations on past events and/or anticipatory worries about what will happen in the future. Focusing on the present moment allows no space for these judgments.

6. On a related note, what feelings do you associate with each of these thoughts? Do you notice any patterns? Are your thoughts about the past or the future more likely to be associated with negative feelings, such as anger, frustration, sadness, or worry?

7. Last, choose one of your identified judgmental thoughts. For the next minute, imagine what it would feel like if you were to let that judgmental thought go. In other words, if you were to just sit with that thought and not try to change it or make it go away. How does it feel to just sit with this discomfort? There are times when we are not able to change a particularly negative or judgmental thought, and the ability to accept the thought for what it is may be the healthiest way to break the hold such thoughts can have over us.

8. Now choose one of your most positive, uplifting thoughts. Take a moment to feel gratitude for this thought. It's important to note these small moments of gratitude every day, so that we don't always pay attention to the negative!

Activity 3: Learn to Engage with Authentic Care

For this exercise, you will practice becoming aware of at least a few of your most cherished personal values. These are typically transcendent values, meaning that they are qualities of self, life, or relationships such as *honesty, love, faith, discipline, sense of mastery and accomplishment in the world* rather than actions, activities, or roles. You will want to find a quiet place to sit, as you did for skill area #1, and you will need a notebook or journal and a pen nearby.

   Imagine that you are nearing the end of your life and are reflecting back on what you learned, appreciated, and valued. Once you can imagine this, bring into your mind qualities of life, yourself, and experiences that you hold most dear. What comes to mind? What scenes do you see? What feelings do you feel? From this inner, centered state, ask yourself what you see that you have really valued and worked hard to cultivate in your life and yourself. Record these in your journal. These are important because they are likely similar to the values you are likely to want your child to cherish as well. It is useful to both keep these in mind and to communicate their importance to your child.

Section 4

Practical Matters

11

Positive Communications During Challenging Times

Dealing with Authority Issues, Power Struggles, and Staying Calm when Your Child Is Not

Each day of our lives we make deposits in the memory banks of our children.

—Charles R. Swindoll

I have grown as a person, a mother, a wife, a teacher because of this experience. I am able to hold myself and my daughter accountable for our interactions and accept that neither one of us can be perfect. She consistently tells others how lucky she is to have parents who love and support her. I take great pride in those comments.

—Faith, mother of a child who self-injures

How many times have you wished that your child could simply and calmly state how she was feeling, where those feelings came from, and what she thought you could do to help? In fact, how many of us have wished that full-grown adults in our lives could do this? As we have touched on in a variety of ways throughout this book, human beings, especially when they are young, use a variety of strategies for communicating what they feel and even what they think, even when they are unable to clearly translate these into words. Self-injury is one such form of communication. And it can be extremely effective in expressing—in physical ways—emotions that defy easy expression otherwise. In general, people who use self-injury to express or manage feelings often have a strong urge to communicate—to themselves, to the world, and, in all likelihood to you—despite their struggle to verbally articulate what they're feeling.

This chapter is devoted specifically to verbal communication because what we say and how we say it are together such a critical part of healthy relationships and family life. Here you will find strategies for using spoken language in effective and supportive ways, for knowing when to engage and when to pull back and bide your time, and how to avoid common power struggles and conflict.

Adolescent Communication 101: Understanding the Language of Youth

Rare is the adolescent or young adult (or adult, for that matter!) who can calmly, clearly, and articulately share the substance of a feeling, identify the thoughts associated with that feeling, talk about where it may have come from, and then seek support or guidance on what to do. This is difficult for almost everyone and is reflected in the fact that humans have many different ways of speaking without words. While clear communication can be difficult for all of us, the very nature of adolescence and young adulthood makes matching up words with feelings very challenging. Indeed, self-injury itself is often an indicator that someone is struggling with intense and complex emotions without being able to easily translate them into words.

As we have alluded to elsewhere, from about the ages of 11 to 25 humans undergo profound developmental change, much of which is unseen. These changes do not happen all at once, but in sometimes confusing fits and starts over time. Indeed, it can take more than a decade before the brain is fully developed in the areas of long-term planning and decision-making. Before then, however, it is very common for teens to believe they are largely immune to long-term negative consequences. Your teen is likely to believe that the consequences of risky behaviors won't happen to her. She's likely to spend more time thinking about what she feels and thinks, and to believe that other people are overwhelmingly focused on what she is doing, thinking, and feeling. Interestingly, despite her keen focus on her own emotions, brain development during the early and middle adolescent years actually makes it harder for individuals to clearly recognize and relate to others' feelings or to take others' perspectives. This intense self-focus can lead to significant drama and absolute certainty that no one on the planet has ever felt just the way that she has.

While it may feel otherwise at times, natural adolescent development is a parent's ally. Over time, it will become easier and easier for young people to identify and recognize feelings and to communicate directly, particularly if they have role models for doing this (this is especially important for males since they are often actively discouraged from showing and articulating their feelings). However, this process can take a long time. It is not uncommon, as you may have experienced first-hand, for teenagers to stop communicating altogether (or perhaps only through grunts or very cryptic statements) or to change from a once-communicative and connective child into someone who seems to have very little to say, very little interest in connection.

> It is important to note that despite how uncommunicative children themselves may seem, they are actually strongly neurologically primed to notice and record even subtle patterns in how adults, particularly those closest to them, communicate.

Despite what it feels like, the seeming lack of communication can, in fact, communicate a lot. The problem is that it's very difficult to tell what exactly the message is! Many parents feel they must be mind-readers during this time, and they do tend to become much more attuned to subtle changes in mood or gesture. It is important to note that despite how uncommunicative children themselves may seem, they are actually strongly neurologically primed to notice and record even subtle patterns in how adults, particularly those closest to them, communicate.

It's fascinating, really, because it seems like they're not paying attention at all. But they are picking up on how you say things, the way you say them, and subtle variations in your tone, facial features, and gestures while you speak. This is not entirely conscious on their part. Because they are deeply absorbed in learning how to be adults, adults around them become focal points for study. As adults, we represent their future, of sorts, but they have little of the certainty we feel (e.g., maybe you have a job or other full-time occupation, some degree of respect from others, can pay bills and take care of problems). You are intensely interesting to your teen in ways that may surprise you and will certainly surprise him if he ever becomes aware of how closely he is watching!

Staying Calm When Your Child Is Not: Managing Conflict by Using the Language of Partnership and Authenticity

Over and over again, we have heard from parents about the doors that have been opened by opening their minds—and hearts—to more effective, positive, healthy communications with their children. These may be hard-won moments, but they can and do happen, often as a by-product of facing the challenges presented by self-injury and related issues over time. Two parents of self-injuring youth had this to say:

> We no longer fear talking about things openly. Nothing is off limits. I've learned not to judge or want to control her.
> —*Mwenda, parent of daughter who self-injures*

The most important thing to know during this time is to *take the long view*. This means trusting that being heard, understood, and getting what you want in each exchange with your child matters less than the cumulative effects of your communication across time. While you want to be heard, understood, and respected—and these are very important for maintaining family balance and harmony—the even bigger task at hand is to show your child what it feels and looks like to be consistent, balanced, and fundamentally respectful and relatable over time. In some cases, this will mean that you will walk away from an interaction with your child feeling unheard, possibly disrespected, or even deeply concerned about your success as a parent. But, if you were able to maintain your cool, convey your point honestly and clearly, and believe that you are coming from a place of love for your child and yourself, then know that you did not likely lose anything in the exchange, and, in all likelihood, you have advanced your cause.

Walking away with some degree of calm also provides an example of healthy coping in the face of adversity. One of the most important things a parent can do is clearly demonstrate effective ways for dealing with hard emotions and/or negative thought patterns. As we have discussed, a growing body of research supports the idea that individuals who use self-injury to manage their emotions do so because they physically experience their emotions much more potently than does the average person due to neurological and physiological predispositions. They are also likely to interpret things in a negative light and be resistant to more positive ways of interpreting or feeling events. In some cases, one or more of their parents will have similar tendencies. Because of this, learning to communicate and speak about hard feelings can be rewarding—for both parents and their children.

> One of the most important things a parent can do is clearly demonstrate effective ways for dealing with hard emotions and/or negative thought patterns.

Tips and Techniques for Building Positive, Healthy Communications

Enhancing your ability to talk and listen to your child is not only important for helping to end self-injury behavior; it is also a valuable tool for all interactions with your child. Here are some important tips and techniques you can use to actively listen and mindfully communicate with your child.

Set Clear Communication Intentions

Not everything uncomfortable or imperfect needs to be fixed, at least not right away. Use the intention clarification exercises in the previous chapter to become clear about what is your highest priority now or later (you can use the exercises regularly as things shift) and focus on the top 2–4 issues that emerge for you. Try to think of problems that seem to be recurring, rather than a single event that may have upset you. For instance, here's an example of how setting clear intentions may play out in real life:

> Sarah was often aggravated at her son Nick, who had recently been ignoring her requests and not following through on things that he said he would do. Sarah could choose to focus on one of these particular events, but she may find it more useful to consider the underlying issue(s) that are recurring over and over. Why are they so upsetting to her? In this case, the larger issue may be a general lack of respect for house rules, or perhaps Sarah feels a bit threatened and perceives Nick as not respecting her as a parent. Before having a conversation with Nick, it is important for Sarah to set a goal for herself for what she wants to discuss with Nick. She may want to focus on the past couple of weeks of ignoring chores and requests, or she may want to focus on Nick's patterns of behavior that suggest a general lack of respect.

> SARAH: "Nick, over the past couple of weeks, I've noticed that you've been late for your curfew and have not followed through on your weekly chores. I can't help but feel as though you are not respecting our house rules and not respecting my role as a parent. This leaves me feeling frustrated and hurt."
>
> NICK: "Mom, I am not doing anything on purpose! I just have a lot going on and can't always get the things done that you ask me to do."
>
> SARAH: "I understand that we all can be pulled in a lot of directions at certain times. If you're feeling like you're not able to get things done around here because of other demands you have at work or at school, then let me know and we can figure out a work-around. I'm happy to do that. But, in order to make all of this work, I have to hear from you what you

need, and you need to show me that you're respecting our house rules. Can you do that?"

NICK: "Yeah, I guess."

SARAH: "Nick, this is important to me so I am going to be watching closely, okay? I will definitely make a point of telling you when you are making good on our agreement, but I'd like to suggest that we see how it goes over the next week or two and touch base again. If you are letting it slip and we need to revisit it all, then I want to know that we have agreed on a time to talk about it. Does that work for you?"

NICK: "Yeah, whatever."

SARAH (NOTING BUT PURPOSEFULLY NOT ENGAGING WITH HIS SLIGHTLY SNARKY TONE): "Great, thanks for agreeing to this. I like knowing that we will have a more formal time to check in; it will keep me from nagging you."

In addition to being very clear about what she wanted and working hard to explain how important his follow-through was to her (as opposed to making accusations about general failings), Sarah was wise to set up a time to revisit the issue. This gives both of them the opportunity to reset and try again, but it also underscores for Nick the importance his mother places on him following through. Sarah should try to note when Nick does follow-through over the next two weeks and tell him how much it means to her.

As an issue or situation is resolved, revised, or parked until another time, you can revisit your primary issues and reorder or replace the focus. If you are not clear about what you want to convey, then it is typically better to wait on starting a conversation until you are more clear. This can be challenging work, and some may find it useful to work on these issues with a therapist.

Set the Stage

Actively listening means you are giving your full attention to the person you are communicating with, making eye contact, and, when possible, not doing anything else. So it's important to choose a time and place appropriate for the conversation. Being in a quiet place without interruptions or distractions and having plenty of time for the discussion helps increase the chances your child will be open to sharing and listening. Some may find that a leisurely weekend morning allows the space for these conversations or perhaps the quiet time before bedtime.

Be Mindful of Whether You Want To Win or To Understand

It is normal to want to maintain or exert control, particularly when we feel out of control of other big things in life, like our child's behaviors or feelings. However, it is also important and useful to let go of winning and instead work to understand both your *and* your child's feelings and perceptions. When in conflict, try to be aware of whether you want to win the argument or to better understand your loved one. Allow your child to have a different point of view from your own—you are trying to engage your child in conversation, this is not a debate. Aiming to understand rather than to be right or heard or have your agenda adopted will facilitate positive communication and help you both understand each other's feelings and perspectives in potentially triggering situations.

> When in conflict, try to be aware of whether you want to win the argument or to better understand your loved one.

For instance, Jessica's daughter Joy had started snapping at Jessica before bed. Jessica was annoyed and wanted it to stop. She realized that her admonishments ("You're not going to talk like that to me, young lady. That's disrespectful!") were not changing much, so she decided to confront Joy directly.

JESSICA: "I am frustrated by your consistently bad mood at night, Joy. Can you help me understand what might be going on for you?"

JOY: "I don't know mom, why don't you just stay away from me if you don't like it so much."

JESSICA NOTED HER TEMPER FLARING AT THIS RESPONSE BUT
SQUASHED HER DESIRE TO DO SOMETHING RASH, LIKE GROUND
JOY FOR HER INSOLENCE. INSTEAD, SHE DECIDED TO REALLY TRY
TO UNDERSTAND. SHE USED THE OBSERVE, DESCRIBE, ENGAGE
APPROACH (SEE CHAPTER 10) TO PAUSE, FIND HER DEEPEST TRUTH
AND SHARE FROM THERE: "Joy, I really love you and I don't
like ending the day with you angry at me. I don't like feeling
disconnected like that. It feels like there's something going on
with you that you're not really sharing. and, because of this,
I feel very helpless like there's nothing I can do for you. Do
you think you could help me understand what's happening
for you?"

From here, the conversation could go in one of many directions,
but it would be surprising if Joy did not soften at least a little and share
something useful and honest with her mother. Jessica reached a critical
juncture at which she realized that if she really wanted to understand,
she'd have to give up on winning. It can be hard to put away the anger
and let go of what feels like rightful parental control in situations like
these, but if you want to understand what's happening for your child
and to help, it behooves a parent to prioritize understanding over winning. If you can do this, you may be amazed by what you come away
with that you did not know before. This strategy opens the door to
ongoing conversation and is likely to make your child more willing to
talk with you in the future, even about difficult topics.

Pay Attention to Nonverbal Communications

As we pointed out earlier, other nonverbal characteristics of communication are important, too. Things like positive tone, sustained eye contact, and facial expressions show you are listening and engaged in the
conversation with your child. Using positive, open gestures (e.g., leaning
forward and nodding) rather than negative ones (e.g., crossing your arms
or putting your hands on your hips) suggest you are listening and open
to the conversation. Although this is not always possible when you are
feeling negative emotions (and this is okay, too—you are human after
all!), it is a good skill to actively work on and to try to model.

Validate Wherever Possible

Have you ever felt frustrated, misunderstood, or isolated? Of course we all have at some point. These are exceptionally common to the adolescent experience. Parents are in a unique and precarious position with their children, in that most children expect that their parents *should* understand in a deep and meaningful way where they are coming from, and yet many parents fail to meet the high bar that has been set for them (or that they set up for themselves). Validation is the skill of actively accepting a person's experience or perspective, in that moment, and communicating that acceptance to them. Simply offering a degree of empathy and understanding of your child's perspectives on life, her feelings and beliefs—no matter how different from yours—and allowing her to see that you appreciate her worldview is empowering and can alter her feelings and behavior.

> Validation is the skill of actively accepting a person's experience or perspective, in that moment, and communicating that acceptance to them.

For example, Lanessa and her daughter, Lara, were in a tough conversation about why Lara had not done the chores Lanessa had asked her to do after school for several days in a row during the previous week. Lara's voice was rising and she knew they were headed for a serious fight. Lanessa decided to simply really listen to Lara and use the validation technique to defuse things and give herself time to figure out what was happening and what to do:

LANESSA: Okay, Lara, our growing frustration with each other makes it clear that we are not really understanding each other. Can you tell me again why you cannot do your chores as we agreed?

LARA: I told you a million times that I am too tired when I get home! You think I am making this up to get out of doing my chores, but I really do not feel well. I have been coming home and sleeping for over an hour every day.

LANESSA: Okay, I hear you saying that you would do the chores if you were feeling well. It also sounds like you are frustrated that I am not really believing that you really are not feeling well.

LARA: Yes! I really have not been feeling well.

LANESSA: I am truly sorry that you are feeling poorly. Let's work on figuring out what is happening for you and we can revisit the chores after that, okay?

LARA: Yes, okay.

Use Deep Listening to Be Sure You Really Understand what You Heard

When you are in the midst of a difficult or frustrating conversation, it helps to use observe, describe, and engage skills to acknowledge your emotions but then focus attention on really listening, with the intention of deeply understanding what is being communicated. You'll want to listen for the feelings as well as to the words. Try to remember that angry words, accusations, and judgments about your character or parenting skills are often camouflage for sadness, hurt, loss, rejection, and other feelings with which you will likely empathize. The hurling of angry words by your child is often meant to protect the softness and vulnerability underneath that he or she may be feeling, by keeping you away from those feelings of sadness or pain (it often works!). But if you listen for what's behind the words, you are likely to detect communication that is gentler and more authentic.

For example, Lateesha had a hard time understanding why her son Daryl was so deeply affected by a recent break up with his girlfriend. Daryl had only been going out with her for a couple of months, and his response to the breakup—becoming despondent, almost never leaving his room, and being profoundly grumpy with everyone—seemed disproportionate to what had happened. Daryl's history of self-injury worried Lateesha but she felt unable to make a connection with him and worried that he was moving into an active self-injury phase. She decided to use the deep listening skills she had recently learned at a workshop, listening for the emotion in Daryl's voice and paying close attention to the particular words he used in order to better understand where he was coming from. Here is how part of that conversation went:

LATEESHA: "Daryl, can you help me understand one more time how you feel about breaking up with Tisha? I really want to understand so that I can support you better. I know you told me before why it hurts so much, but I wonder if you could share with me one more time so I can work on listening and understanding better?"

DARYL: "Oh mom, I don't know if I want to talk about it anymore. It's like I already told you, she just got under my skin. I don't even know—we were hanging out and everything is great and the next day she's breaking up with me. It's over, and I'm over it, okay!? I just don't want to have it happen again."

LATEESHA (THIS TIME WHEN SHE LISTENED, SHE REALIZED SHE COULD FEEL THE HURT IN HER SON'S VOICE. BUT, MORE THAN THAT, SHE FELT THE INTENSITY IN WHAT HE HAD LAST SAID: "I don't want to have it happen again." She wondered if this was somehow connected to a big fight he and his dad got into last year. They hadn't talked to each other since. She suddenly had a hunch that the two experiences were connected, so she decided to check it out): "Okay, so what I hear is a lot of sadness, a sense of rejection by somebody that you thought really understood you. It felt so sudden, didn't it? It seems like it took you off guard and that was very painful. Is any of that right?"

DARYL: "Yeah—it just felt so sad and I really didn't have any idea. I thought it was going so well."

LATEESHA: "I'm going to go out on a limb here, Daryl, but I wonder if when you said "I really don't want to have it happen again" you might've been feeling the same feelings that you had when you and your dad had that big fight last year. I remember you saying it felt sudden, that you weren't sure what happened—a lot of the same words. I know it's been hard for you not to see him for so long. I wonder if this feels kind of like both of them just dropped you. If so, I can imagine that thinking about both Tisha and your dad would feel big and bad. Am I on target at all?"

DARYL (AFTER A PAUSE): "Yeah, maybe. I've been thinking about that a lot and I feel really angry at him, too. I dunno . . . it's just all so dark right now."

Lateesha left the conversation feeling much more in tune with what was happening for Daryl. She could not fix it, but her understanding and compassion meant Daryl felt less alone. In addition, she was able to provide him the space he needed to process the feelings he was having. He told her that he had felt like cutting, but he had not done it so far. He agreed to tell her if he started to feel like he could not resist the urge and seemed grateful that she understood.

> Deep listening is most easily accomplished if our own emotions are calm and centered, but it is nearly impossible if they are running high.

Deep listening is a powerful technique since it is really about listening for the underlying, often unspoken emotion in someone's words, tone, and body language. It is most easily accomplished if our own emotions are calm and centered, but it is nearly impossible if they are running high. After listening to what has been said, you can comment or ask questions about what you just heard to be sure you understood. It helps to be specific about the situation even when the person speaking is making global statements (e.g., using words like "never" or "always"). If you're not sure you are getting the full meaning, you can also state, in your own words, what you think you heard. You can start this by saying something like "So what I hear you saying is. . . . " It is especially powerful if you can translate into words the feelings that you think you hear your child conveying to you. If you can summarize what you think you're hearing on an emotional level without making a declarative statement about what you *believe* you're hearing, it can be very validating. This kind of reflective listening helps your child feel heard and helps you understand his or her message. Asking questions can also keep the conversation going.

Take a Break If You Need It

If things are becoming uncomfortable or either one of you is feeling overwhelmed, you can say so and suggest continuing the conversation at another time. Keep in mind that you can always come back to a difficult conversation, even if you feel you didn't handle it the way you wanted to the first time. Allow the same for your child. Similarly, if a difficult conversation quickly turns negative or ends poorly, give yourself and your child permission to have the discussion another time. It's okay for you to acknowledge to your child that you wish you had responded differently as a way of opening the conversation. Many parents wish the first conversation with their child about self-injury had gone differently. Understand that although it may sometimes feel like it, the door has *not* closed on this conversation. Acknowledging that you felt it didn't go well can show your child that you want to talk more about it and that you are working to make future conversations more positive. This is also particularly potent because it models to your child a strategy for coming back around to a hard topic. Learning how to be vulnerable is tough for everyone, and kids need to watch adults do that in order to try it out themselves.

Be Creative with Means of Communication

Not all communication has to be face-to-face, particularly in the modern age. Maybe you can more easily communicate via texts, written notes left for each other, or in emails. Sometimes the car—where eye contact is not an expectation and no one can leave—can be a good place for a conversation. Although this removes the possibility for eye contact (one of the characteristics of active listening), talking in the car might actually be easier when discussing sensitive or embarrassing topics. A series of short conversations spread out over days or weeks might work better than one long discussion. There is no one "right way" to communicate with your child—use the method that works best for the two of you.

Be as Authentic as Possible

The most critical advice we can give you is to be as authentic as possible in your communications. This means taking the time to figure out what you honestly feel and think and then finding a way to communicate that as honestly as possible. This goes for negative as well as positive feelings. For example, when a child is acting in ways that frustrate, anger, or hurt you, you can find a way to state this authentically but without adding fuel to the proverbial fire by saying something such as:

> I really want to be patient and to try to understand what you're telling me right now, but it feels like you're accusing me and, perhaps,

acting out your anger on me. I know you're having a lot of feelings you can't control right now, but it's hard for me to be fully present for you when this is happening. How about you say whatever else you need to say and I'll take a little time to think about it all and come back to you when I'm not feeling so triggered.

Being authentic may also mean that you share vulnerability, "wearing your feelings on your sleeve" as they say, and this can be kind of scary. After all, who wants to feel rejected after you put yourself out there? Pausing to figure out your feelings, particularly if you feel yourself getting angry, irritated, or otherwise reactive, helps with being as authentic as possible.

Here's another example of what authenticity might look like as conveyed to your child:

> I sometimes feel really helpless with all of this, like it is bigger than me and even us or our family. It makes me feel scared and like I am failing. I want to connect with you, to be together in this, but right now I feel at a loss about how to do that. I really want to work together to figure out how to do this differently. Do you want this, too?

It is very likely that you will feel much calmer after stating this truth in a way that does not blame your child. "I statements" are an incredibly useful way of helping you get to core feelings and beliefs at the root of the issue at hand and allow you to share authentic, meaningful communications. It also helps to not catastrophize or generalize (e.g., avoid use of the words "always" and "never" or any equivalent that suggests a permanent hopelessness). If you can do these things with any regularity, you will also have shown your child how to be vulnerable but articulate and honest at the same time; this is a difficult but immensely valuable skill to model.

In your pursuit of authenticity, it helps to try to move yourself beyond the tendency to frame your feelings entirely in terms of what the other person is doing and figure out *why* it bothers you so much. What inside of you, in your background or current life, is being needled? It can be helpful to ask yourself "where and when have I felt like this in the past?" What is the earliest memory you can find? (For example, "ah—I get it . . . when my child yells that I suck as a parent, I automatically feel like I used to feel as a child when my father scowled and told me that I was making his life difficult.")

> If you need to take time or ask for a pause while you tune into your own cascade of feelings or associations, take it.

It can help to use the observe, describe, engage strategy here to help you figure out what is going on before responding to your child. If you need to take time or ask for a pause while you tune into your own cascade of feelings or associations, take it.

Remember, modeling these things is helpful for your child. Intense reactions are often simply triggering memories of other times, perhaps of when you were younger and more vulnerable. Understanding this can reduce some of the intensity that may be interfering with your ability to understand and respond to the present situation.

Putting It Together: Examples of Positive and Not So Positive Communications

Here are two different scenarios in which a parent, Jim, interacts with his daughter, Anna, when she comes home after her curfew. See if you can figure out what skills and tools Jim uses in the more successful scenario in comparison to the less successful scenario (you can figure that one out on your own, too!).

Scenario 1

As Jim waited for Anna to come home, he could feel his frustration and anger growing. He wanted to go to bed, and he had acquiesced to letting Anna stay out so late against his best judgment. She had promised to be home by now. When she came in more than an hour late, the conversation started:

> JIM: "Where have you been? I have been waiting for over an hour! You promised that you would be home on time if I let you go out. I knew I shouldn't have let you go out! Where have you been?"
>
> ANNA: "Jeez, dad, why are you freaking out?!! I'm not that late, and it wasn't my fault!"
>
> JIM: (takes a breath and gathers himself) "Anna, I get worried when you are out late and when I cannot contact you. I tried

texting you but received no response. Plus, I am really tired and want to sleep. I cannot do that when I know you are out, especially these days."

ANNA: "What do you mean by 'especially these days??' You never listen to me! I told you where I was, and it wasn't my fault that I was late coming home—it was Kara's fault because she couldn't find her keys. You never trust me and always think I am doing bad things when I am not!"

JIM: (feeling even more frustrated and tired, raises his voice) "This has nothing to do with trust, it has to do with worrying about you. And, yes, 'especially these days' is because we are all worried about you, about you cutting again. That has really affected the family, Anna, and it doesn't feel like you understand that at all. You need to start taking more responsibility here!"

ANNA: (defensiveness increasing) "I cannot believe you are saying this! I have been very responsible, and I haven't cut in a few weeks and it was *not* my fault! My phone died so I could not text you back, and we were all outside searching high and low for Kara's keys in the dark that I didn't think about borrowing a phone. I was sure we would find them and then I would be home. You always blame me!!" (Stomps off to her room and slams the door.)

It is hard to say where this would go from here exactly, but we can safely assume that neither Anna nor Jim (and perhaps other members of house awakened by the yelling and slamming) slept soundly that night. Moreover, it is likely that the chill with which they ended the conversation persisted and, perhaps, led to increased tension. Take a few minutes to think about what Jim might have done to leave things in a different state. Where did he use the strategies we have been discussing, and where could he have done better?

Scenario 2

As Jim waited for Anna to come home, he could feel his frustration and anger growing. He wanted to go to bed, and he had acquiesced to letting Anna stay out so late over his better judgment. She had promised to be home by now. When she came in more than an hour late, the conversation started:

JIM: "Where have you been? I have been waiting for over an hour! You promised that you would be home on time if I let you go out. I knew I shouldn't have let you go out! Where have you been?"

ANNA: "Jeez, dad, why are you freaking out?!! I'm not that late and it wasn't my fault!"

JIM: (takes a breath and gathers himself. He is about to tell Anna how irresponsible she has been, but stops himself. He knew he wasn't in a good state of mind to have a conversation. He pauses and then says) "Anna, we are both tired and should sleep before we talk more. I really want both of us to understand each other, and we cannot do that well now, so let's sleep now and talk more when we are rested."

ANNA: (she had been prepared for a tirade so was surprised and both a little nervous and relieved) "Okay." She walks off to her room and closes the door gently so as not to wake anyone or risk losing this brief reprieve.

Here is how Jim handled the conversation the next morning:

JIM: "I want to talk about what happened last night. Are you ready to talk now, too?"

ANNA: "I guess so" (stated in a defensive tone). "You never listen to me! I told you where I was, and it wasn't my fault that I was late coming home—it was Kara's fault because she couldn't find her keys. You never trust me and always think I am doing bad things when I am not!"

JIM: (pauses to listen and let it sink in. He is aware of rising defensiveness and a need to make her see how irresponsible he thinks she was, but he knows where that will go. Instead, he works on putting himself in her place and understanding) "Okay, I think I understand your frustration. I hear you saying that you feel like I did not really hear or trust you when you told me that you were trying to come home on time but that you could not do much to make Kara find her keys faster than she did. This made you feel a little powerless and stuck. Am I hearing you right?"

ANNA: (defensiveness subsiding) "Yeah, I guess so. But you always do that."

JIM: "I don't know about always, but I can see that I wasn't listening very well in this case. I was feeling frustrated that you were not home on time, and I wanted to go to sleep and know that you were home safely. I wish that you had texted or called me when Kara realized that she lost her keys and you knew you were going to be late. I felt angry and tired and worried. This makes it hard for me to listen. I promise to work on this. Do you think you can also work on understanding what I might be feeling in these situations, too? Maybe next time you could try to let me know what was happening earlier so I wouldn't worry? I would like for us to work together in situations like this."

From here, the conversation could go in many directions. Take a few minutes to think about what Jim did differently in this scenario than in Scenario 1. Where did he use the strategies we have been discussing?

From our perspective, Jim did much better in the second scenario than in the first because he effectively diffused the tension and opened the door for honest connection with Anna. Since things did not start out well, Jim stopped the conversation and said that he wanted to pick it up in the morning, after a night's rest and some time to allow flaring tempers to calm down. This strategy gave them both space to quiet their emotions before they talked the next morning. When they spoke the next morning, the conversation went much differently than it probably would have the night before. While they were talking about events and behaviors, what was really going on under the surface—which Jim addressed quite well—were the *feelings* they were both having. Both felt frustrated by things out of their control, and nothing they said was actually going to matter until those feelings were recognized. Jim tuned into Anna's underlying feelings, even though Anna did not talk about them explicitly. He also admitted both that he understood her feelings now and that he had not listened nor shared her feelings when she first expressed them. Thus, he validated Anna and himself. This validation opens the door for productive conversation about the specific behaviors and situations that need to be addressed. It is important to note that Jim did not let his child off the hook for being late, but he did model both positive coping and communication and then allowed for authentic sharing.

Your Turn: Using the Tools for Positive, Healthy Communications

The situation: Beth thought that her 16-year-old son, Malik, had stopped injuring and hadn't engaged in it since she first learned about his skin carving several weeks before. So she was shocked to find evidence of recent self-injury. Knowing that she was not in the best emotional state to talk with him at that time and that doing so might lead to accusatory comments driven by anger or frustration ("You promised me that you would come to me when you felt the need to cut your body and talk with me. Why didn't you do that?"), she chose to wait until she had time to think about what she wanted to say.

- What advice would you give Beth to help make the conversation with Malik as productive as possible?
- What advice would you give Beth about setting her communication intentions?

What happened next: Beth asked Malik if they could talk for a few minutes one Saturday afternoon when everyone else in the family was out of the house. Here's how that conversation went:

BETH: "Last week, I found blood in the bathroom. It worried me. I wondered if we could check in with each other to talk about this and see how you're doing?"

MALIK: "How come you assume that it was me injuring myself?" (said defensively)

BETH: "I'm trying not to assume anything, so that's why I'm coming to you about this. In addition to the blood, though, I couldn't help but notice that you have seemed very stressed and irritable over the last several days. I wondered if you may be feeling overwhelmed and triggered."

MALIK: "Well, yes, I have been stressed out. Good of you to notice!" (said sarcastically) "I knew that if I told you, you'd be mad and, like, 'You're what?! Why are you doing that again?!'"

BETH: (pauses for about 10 seconds and takes a couple of breaths, noticing the tension in her chest and realizing that she felt worried that this conversation was going to head south and that it would leave them worse off than before. She decides to share this and uses "I statements" to help her to authentically share with her son) "I can see how you would feel anxious about talking about this and maybe feel like you're letting me—and yourself—down. To be perfectly honest, this is something that's a little scary for me. I not only worry about your well-being but about how to bring this issue up in a way that shows how much I care, and my genuine concern, without making you feel bad or more stressed. I very much want to help you and us, not make things worse."

MALIK (becoming less defensive): "This isn't something you can help with. It's something that I have to deal with on my own."

BETH: "I can imagine that it feels that way. I know how it feels to need to take care of my own problems myself. But, I also know that all of us need help sometimes. I've had to learn that one in some hard ways, too. I'm not here to judge you or to tell you how to live your life. I'm just someone who cares deeply for you and who wants to help you. I need you to know that you are not alone. How can we work together to both support your need to figure out your own problems and also help you feel less alone with it all? You may not feel like sharing everything with me, but it may be helpful to sort out some of what's stressing you with a professional. How do you feel about that? Do you have other ideas about what might help you to help yourself?"

• What positive communication skills did Beth use?

- What did Beth do to observe, describe, and engage in this conversation? What else would you recommend she take into account when using observe, describe, engage?

- Do you think Beth was being authentic in her communications? How might she have been more authentic in her sharing?

- Where do you think the conversation might go from here? What are the possibilities you see based on the exchange so far?

- If this was a conversation that had taken place between you and your child, where do you think the conversation might go from here? How could you imagine working to help ensure that the conversation stays focused, productive, and positive?

Talking About Self-Injury: How to Start the Conversation and Keep the Door Open

The best way to initiate what could be a hard conversation about self-injury in a way likely to keep lines of communication open is to use "respectful curiosity." Respectful curiosity is a state of awareness characterized by a genuine curiosity and willingness to know and understand while ensuring that one's curiosity is satisfied in a kind and respectful way. First coined by Caroline Kettlewell in her 2000 book *Skin Games* and then popularized by Barent Walsh in *Treating Self-Injury: A Practical Guide*, this concept is powerful for parents and others who care for someone who self-injures. Indeed, it is a wonderful parenting technique all around—particularly in times when you feel perplexed about your child's attitude or behavior.

> Respectful curiosity is a wonderful parenting technique all around—particularly in times when you feel perplexed about your child's attitude or behavior.

Since you cannot know what will and will not feel respectful to another person, even your own child, it is wise to obtain permission to ask questions or to preface your questions with an exploratory statement, something like, "I want to do everything I can to help you feel supported and respected. I also want to better understand what you feel, think, and experience. Do you mind if I ask a few questions to help me better understand?"

Even if one or more of your questions is uncomfortable for your child, she is more likely to trust your intentions if you have been clear. Also, your efforts will have the benefit of modeling for your child emotional honesty and clarity. Similarly, it is *very* important to honor your child's responses and disclosures. If she does not want to share something, or anything, you will need to accept this with as much grace and humility as possible—even if it frustrates you or hurts your feelings. Prefacing your question with something that conveys your sincere intention to deeply listen and understand, such as "Can you help me understand?" or "Do you mind if I ask you a question?" can do a lot to minimize defensiveness. If you can couple this opening with an authentic desire to understand what your child communicates, through language and more subtle emotional cues, you may be very surprised at how enjoyable it can be to have these conversations. Even though the content is difficult, the subtle emotional exchange happening between the two of you can feel immensely gratifying and can set the stage for continuing discussion. Here are a few examples of respectfully curious questions specific to self-injury:

"Can you help me understand . . ."

- "Why self-injury works so well for you?"
- "How it makes you feel emotionally afterward?"
- "What kinds of feelings or experiences make you want to self-injure?"
- "Are there particular emotions that make you want to self-injure?"
- "What are some reasons it feels hard to stop?"
- "What happened with this slip? You've been successful in not self-injuring before—what do you think was different this time?"
- "What I can do to support you?"
- "What kinds of things I do, or what happens in our family, that triggers you?"

Since listening with an open heart and mind can be very challenging, particularly if you are hearing negative input about yourself, it can help to take time to distance yourself from your thoughts and/or feelings and simply observe your inner reactions as though you are an outsider looking in or as if you are watching a movie. If you notice that you feel judgmental, angry, or like you want to lash out, this is the time to hit the pause button and come back to the conversation later, when you are calm. You can do this by being honest: "I am glad you are sharing all of this with me, and I do want to hear it all. However, I am having a hard time hearing it all at once, so I want to take a little break, okay? Can we come back to this in a half hour or so [time frame for revisiting can be set by you, but try not to wait too long]? I think I will be able to hear you better if I can sit for a while with what you have already shared."

> If you notice that you feel judgmental, angry, or like you want to lash out, this is the time to hit the pause button.

If you have feelings that you can respectfully and calmly share, then it is helpful to use "I" statements. Here are some examples of these that may help you with listening and responding with composure:

- "I am sorry if I seem uncomfortable with some of this—it is hard for me to know that you hurt."
- "I am so glad that we are finally talking about this; I have felt worried about it for a while but have not known what to say."
- "I feel sad and sometimes worried that something I have done is making you want to hurt yourself."
- "This scares me because I don't know what to do or how to help you."
- "I am starting to feel upset and think I need to take a little space. I want to know more, though, and will let you know when I am ready."
- "If you don't want to talk to me about this now, I understand. I just want you to know that I am here for you when you decide you are ready to talk. Is it okay if I check in with you about this, or would you prefer to come to me?"

Remember to thank your child (and yourself!) for confronting something so difficult and challenging. Since self-injury is a way of *speaking* strong emotion, actually using words to honestly share feelings can be very powerful and healing.

Think Short Conversations, Not "the Big Conversation"

Nutritionists often recommend that we eat several small meals every day rather than one larger meal. This is because it is easier for our bodies to digest and use nutrients in smaller doses. Similarly, the "stuff" of conversations, whether sharing perspectives, facts, stories, emotions, or lessons, is often best digested in small doses. Not only does this make it easier to understand all that is being conveyed, but it builds a much stronger foundation for future exchanges. It is not uncommon for parents of self-injuring youth to have several, short, heart-to-heart conversations about what is happening on a daily, weekly, or monthly basis and to feel quite deeply connected as a result. This is powerful and often cathartic and even healing. The trick is to continually find opportunities for sharing feelings or questions that feel difficult, tender, or otherwise vulnerable. Here are a few tips for accomplishing this:

- *If a door is open—even a little bit—walk through.* Sometimes we just know that someone is a little more open and willing than usual. If you sense it and have been wanting to ask or share something, and the time and place support it (e.g., privacy can be respected), then take advantage of this rather than waiting for the "perfect" time (since there is no such thing).
- *Pick one or two questions or perspectives to share (not four, five, or twenty).* Take a minute to think about what is most important right now, how to frame it respectfully while still being authentic, and focus on that. Have faith that another door will open before long.
- *If you have things to share or ask, make a space for conversation.* Finding time to have a real conversation with one another can be more challenging now than ever, given the many competing demands for our time and attention. That's why it's so important that you set aside a time during which you can talk with one another and not have interference from devices or other family members. This means carefully considering both a time and a place. If home is chaotic or doesn't offer much privacy, perhaps a walk in the neighborhood may be better or a drive to a local ice cream shop. Set the stage and then move forward, even if you feel unsure. Again though, less is generally more in terms of the content of what you should plan to convey. We all do better when we have less to chew on and digest at a time.
- *Keep your hopes realistic.* Tender and cathartic moments can feel great and can make a difference in what happens next. But they rarely "fix" the problem or change anyone enough to radically alter a habit or family dynamic. These moments are more like raindrops that eventually accumulate and create puddles, lakes, and oceans. These positive moments do add up, but meaningful changes take some time and patience.

- *Use some of these small openings to share gratitude or appreciations for the changes you do see.* Take advantage of opportunities to simply share something light, loving, and/or appreciative. This makes a *huge* difference in the quality of a relationship. This is true for all relationships and can play a powerful and transformative role in the life of someone who is struggling with emotional and mental health challenges.

Dealing with Power Struggles

Power struggles with parents and adults in authority are a normal part of adolescent development since it is during this time of life that young people are beginning to express independence and autonomy. Adolescents are more willing to question authority—especially their parents'. Power struggles pose unique challenges for parents and other adults working with youth who self-injure. Many parents fear that setting rules (e.g., curfews, punishments) may contribute to acting out by self-injuring, and this fear generates confusing and difficult feelings.

> The best way to avoid a power struggle is to simply not engage in one. The moment you realize that the struggle is starting is the moment to begin disengaging.

How do you know when a power struggle is happening? A power struggle begins when your child refuses to do something you ask, follow a rule you have set, or participate in activities in which he or she is expected to join. Many times the resistance has less to do with the specific request and more to do with simply wanting to exercise control or power. It is *very* easy to take the bait as parents or other concerned adults, particularly when what we believe we are asking is reasonable or has already been agreed on. While it is virtually impossible to avoid all power struggles, adults can minimize them by staying aware of a few basic strategies.

Strategy 1: Disengage Early

The best way to avoid a power struggle is to simply not engage in one. The moment you realize that the struggle is starting is the moment to begin disengaging. This is not about giving in. What do we mean by "disengaging" from the power struggle? It is about taking the time and space you need to figure out how to manage your child's resistance while you are calm and not overwhelmed by strong emotions. If your child is becoming argumentative, it helps to keep your tone and voice calm and even. If you feel your emotions starting to rise, work on acknowledging and accepting your feelings without reacting impulsively. Remember: *you have time.* In most cases, you can revisit things later. You can also let your child vent or exhaust his negative feelings without reacting in kind. Let your child know that you are not ignoring him, but that you are just listening and want to take time to think about it all. Remember, it takes two to fight; you can simply decide that you will not participate. Then, when you have collected your thoughts and your emotions are in check, you can return to the conversation and calmly discuss the issue using the positive communication skills we discussed earlier in this chapter.

Strategy 2: Create Win–Win Situations

When you are calm, try asking yourself how you might both get something you want from the situation. What do you see as non-negotiable, and where would you be willing to compromise in order to get what is really important to you? Be clear with yourself and then, when you are ready, talk with your child. Give him options for achieving what he wants while also being clear about what is important to you. This can allow for developing a workable middle ground in which everyone achieves something they want. Also, if your child has a choice between options for when and how he can meet the obligations that you are proposing, he has more autonomy and decision-making abilities and will be more likely to accept the framework you're proposing as acceptable. Not all issues carry the same amount of importance and flexibility. Family curfews, for example, may not be flexible. You could, however, offer a small degree of flexibility for special occasions or for weekends versus weeknights. It can be very helpful to let your child know that you are willing to consider different scenarios and that he can be a part of the decision-making. You can likely envision some areas of contention that you are willing to be more flexible with, while others may be harder to compromise on. This will vary from family to family.

Strategy 3: Collaboration

Try thinking of your child as a partner in the negotiation process. It can be helpful to create opportunities for conversations about what is important to each of you *during times in which you are both calm and able to talk*. The goal of these conversations can be to come to agreements about what you each expect and need from one another—and consequences if these expectations are not met. This could be specific to self-injurious behavior, such as expectations about self-injury practices and tools, or it could relate to other issues likely to trigger intense emotions for the parent or child. Having clear, *agreed-upon* consequences for not fulfilling a responsibility can also help circumvent an argument or power struggle or at least help to guide the next steps when consequences become necessary. In the example earlier, for example, Jim and Anna could continue their discussion about consequences for Anna's lateness. Just because Jim dedicated himself to understanding Anna's position does not mean that he will not want there to be consequences. In this case, however, he could suggest a consequence that enhances their or their family's connection, and, ideally, he will ask Anna to help him come up with good ideas for this (e.g., perhaps Anna will agree to attend a family function she was not interested in or will go to a movie with her parents instead of out with a friend). Involving Anna in the decision about what a natural (and hopefully beneficial) consequence might look like can yield great benefits for everyone.

Strategy 4: Use Positive Consequences for Misbehavior

When we think of setting up consequences or punishment for unacceptable behavior or as a strategy for helping to shape and guide new, more desirable behaviors in our children, we most commonly think of taking things away (e.g., screen time) or restricting freedom (e.g., time with friends, activities). As an alternative, consider using "positive consequences" instead. In general, positive consequences are activities that help build needed skills, reduce isolation, and/or engender positive feelings between your child and others in their world. Positive consequences commonly include forms of service or support for others. Examples could include community service, helping a sibling with homework or a neighbor or family member with a household project, or helping to clean up the kitchen after dinner. In this way, the consequence can do "double duty"—serving as a reminder of the misbehavior but also helping to shape new skills and habits. Referring to these consequences at the start of a power struggle, reminding your young person that he or she took part in defining them, and consistently holding him or her accountable for his or her actions can help stop—or at least more quickly calm—a power struggle.

Strategy 5: Patience and Persistence

Keep in mind that these kinds of struggles are normal and are actually a sign of a child's healthy development and growing independence. Figuring out how to make room for your child's developing autonomy, independence, and limit-testing in a way that does not create conflict is something you can work on together. There will likely be moments when you feel like you are failing or when it seems like, no matter how reasonable you are, your child will take the path of *most resistance* rather than least. As one parent, Shelly, notes, "Learning to cope and parent a child with self-injury is *hard work*. It takes a long time and progress is very slow. Fear about the outcome/future and guilt about parenting mistakes (divorce, feeling invalidated) are hard to live with."

> Remember to acknowledge yourself and your child for getting through hard situations with *any* grace.

Strategy 6: Gratitude

Remember to acknowledge yourself and your child for getting through hard situations with *any* grace. Every little reminder of a job well done is good for everyone—even if it is not a job done perfectly. When was the last time you showed yourself or others some gratitude? This can never be overdone.

Activity

Putting It Together

Think back over the past week or two and consider a tough issue that has come up between you and your child, one that brings up some difficult emotions for you, but that you're willing to share and talk about with your child. For instance, this could mean a discussion about how she is managing her experience of strong emotions or her ambivalence about self-injury. Don't feel that you must begin straight away with a highly emotionally charged issue for the two of you; start off gradually so that you each can develop these skills and meet with some success.

For this activity, we would like you to find a time to sit down with your child and share your feelings about this particular issue in order to work toward the goal of authentic sharing, deep listening, and respectful curiosity. This is not about winning or "getting your point across," which implies a one-sided conversation. The goal of this conversation is not to "solve the problem," although you will find that by simply sharing and learning, you're one step closer to solving an underlying problem or issue. It can be helpful to keep a journal handy to record responses to the following questions or just to record general impressions after the conversation ends.

The following steps are designed to help you with navigating this conversation, along with some pointers to keep in mind as you prepare. Here are a few things to do and keep in mind as you prepare for this activity.

PREPARING FOR THE CONVERSATION

1. *Think of an issue you would like to discuss with your child.*

2. *What is your intention/goal in discussing this issue (in other words, what would you like to accomplish with this conversation?):* Practice by writing down here some of your thoughts and feelings on this particular issue that you would like to share with your child. Remember that this is about sharing and understanding each other's feelings and perspectives on this issue.

3. *Set the time and place:* Consider a time when you (and your child) are not likely to be stressed, rushed for time, or distracted by others. Keep in mind that conversations such as these do not necessarily require a lot of time.

4. *What respectfully curious questions can you imagine asking your child about how you may be able to help her with managing this issue?* Remember to practice deep, mindful listening and respectful curiosity. These strategies will serve as powerful tools to help with answering your questions. Avoid using "why" questions. Instead, use "how" questions to explore their sentiments more deeply and touch on your child's thoughts, feelings, and intentions.

5. *Apply mindful parenting strategies.* Practicing openness, empathy, and being nonjudgmental can be incredibly challenging as it requires staying in the present moment and "listening between the lines" of the words your child is saying. What mindful parenting skills did you use well? Which ones would you like to incorporate next time?

6. *Keep your expectations in check. Don't set the bar too high for success!* If your conversation lasts only 2 minutes, but it's a mindful, present conversation that doesn't end in someone stomping out of the room, then consider it a success.

REFLECTING ON THE CONVERSATION

1. *How did you do? Review and notice patterns.* Once you've had a hard conversation, be honest with yourself and assess how you think it went. What did you do well? What could you have done better? What would you want to work on for next time?

2. *What negative thoughts and judgments did you notice?* Reflect on any negative thoughts you may have noticed creeping into your head, either during the conversation or after you finished. How might you challenge or reframe these?

3. *Reflect on the content of the conversation.* Look past the words your child used and consider the feelings behind them. What else was she communicating to you in addition to words?

At first, try this exercise during a time when things are emotionally calm between the two of you. As you develop your listening skills, you will be able to remain in the moment, to listen to words being said and the meaning behind them, in order for you to be more mindful of the connection between the two of you. These strategies are meant to strengthen and develop your relationship with your child and also to support your child's growing need for independence and aid you both in stretching your abilities to express your emotions in a positive manner. Remember, it's never about a single conversation cure-all, but a series of small conversations that can provide bits of learning and understanding that are immensely beneficial to healing and growing for all.

A Few Other Things to Keep in Mind

While you may feel that you're often working at odds with your child, let's face it: for better or worse, you and your child are a team, working alongside one another through the challenges you face in managing strong emotions and self-harm thoughts and behaviors. Your actions during chaotic and challenging times have enormous impact. How do we get through these times and learn from them so that the problem doesn't happen again? And perhaps also make something good come out of it so that we are better off? How do you rise to this challenge as a leader?

Nancy Koehn, a historian at the Harvard Business School, has studied the qualities of leaders who are effective in times of crisis. Considering that we are all leaders of many aspects of our lives (or at least perceived as such by our children, spouses, elderly parents, etc.), Koehn offers a recipe of sorts for living well and cultivating personal growth in order to communicate more effectively and to better understand, appreciate, and support those we love. There is a meaningful parallel here between what she identifies as core qualities of effective leaders in crisis and what we have seen in parents who successfully navigate the difficulties that come with having a child who is struggling in some significant way. Historically, effective leaders:

- have awareness of their emotions and how they contribute to a situation;
- try not to personalize the situation, understanding that the situation is not directed at them and is not a direct reflection of their abilities;
- reflect on and learn from what's happening inside and around them so that they're better prepared down the road;
- consider others' perspectives not as barriers to their own success but as opportunities for growth; and
- ask themselves, during difficult times, what can be learned and use what they learn to work toward preventing difficulties from happening again.

Application of these leadership qualities to parenting a child who is self-injuring yields a few important messages:

- *Be aware of your emotions and the thoughts driving them*: No matter how well you may think you hide your emotions, your family likely has some sense of what's under the surface. Awareness of these emotions, challenging those negative thoughts and irrational beliefs, and coming to terms with where things stand with a difficult situation will only make you stronger for yourself and your loved ones.

- *You are not a victim, you are an active agent in your life*: Hopefully, this book has given you opportunities to understand and discover your strength, resilience, and focus. The cognitive-behavioral skills and mindful parenting and communication techniques discussed are tools that will help you to work through these difficult days.

- *You can—and should—ask for and receive support*: You are not alone. Concern for one's child and wanting to assure that he has the support he needs is often a parent's primary concern. Parents need to lean on their support systems—informal (friends and family) and formal (therapy)—to be sure that they are taking care of themselves as well.

- *You can use your struggle to grow stronger and to assist others.* Having a child who is struggling, especially if he faces multiple challenges, can definitely strain inner and external resources. But, it can also lead to new perspectives, deeper self-understanding and compassion, and surprisingly often, stronger family bonds. Over and over again we have heard families talk about the strengths they have developed as a result of their experiences with helping their children.

- *You still have responsibilities to the rest of your family*: When a family member seems to be in special need or crisis, all attention tends to turn that way. It is very important for everyone, including your self-injurious child, to know that *all* family members have needs that will require time and attention from you and others.

Establishing Guidelines and Expectations for Managing Self-Injury Behaviors

At first it caused us to hover, shelter, and stifle because we were so scared. We were completely caught off guard. We over compensated, lowered expectations and babied ... most of these things were more detrimental than helpful. In some ways, I feel we got too entangled, I thought I needed to be her support all the time, it was exhausting and a crutch to her. With lots of reading and a good family thera-pist, we learned and are still learning to set appropriate boundaries and to let her learn . . . to stop rescuing her. If she cuts, we didn't cause it, she is learning to deal with her feelings. . . . Boundaries and rules are vital and part of parenting. If you are parenting out of fear and end up lowering the bar for success, you aren't helping your child. We are all learning and growing.

—Tamir, parent of an adolescent who self-injures

The previous chapter focused on communicating compassion and patience as key ingredients of support, but establishing clear boundaries and expectations is important, too. Having clear intentions is helpful in both locating and staying true to your parenting "true north." Study after study shows that clear, calm communications about expectations and consequences are instrumental in healthy family functioning and recovering from difficult times. Determining what you can and cannot tolerate and what you need in order to function with a reasonable degree of balance, as an individual and as a family, is important.

While all families will have to renegotiate expectations and boundaries as children grow into adolescents and then young adults, families with self-injuring youth face unique challenges in this regard. Issues related to wound display in and outside of the house, participating in therapy, school attendance and academics, and other areas of family life that intersect with self-injury are likely to lead to conversations and the need for clearly stated expectations. Moreover, families where self-injury plays a role will have unique needs depending on whether there are siblings in the house and how old the siblings are; how visible the injury patterns are and how they have affected other members of the family in the past; who in the family is and is not aware of the injury; and how emotion, especially intense emotion, is most often handled.[1]

Clearly articulating your expectations and deciding on reasonable consequences if rules are breached is important. Here are some steps to help guide you through this process:

Step 1: *Identify the areas in need of clear policies and expectations.* Have a conversation with any others involved in parenting your child to ensure that you are on the same page and that you have prioritized your concerns in a similar manner.

Step 2: *Identify your "bottom line" requirements.* Think about what you personally and/or others in your family need to be able to co-exist with someone who is injuring. Consider whether you have a "bottom line"—what you absolutely have to have in order to live alongside someone who injures. Examples may include:

- I cannot live with seeing blood around the house.
- I cannot see fresh wounds on my child—it upsets me too much.
- I have to know that my child is home and safe before I go to sleep at night.

Understanding your bottom line requirements will simplify and clarify conversations with your child about these issues and your needs.

> Step 3: *Use effective communication strategies.* Revisit the principles discussed in Chapter 11 concerning effective communication. Reviewing these principles will help you prepare for a conversation about boundaries while maintaining your willingness to understand your child's need to feel safe and in control of her or his life and future. Of utmost importance is maintaining your intention to understand and connect with your child, even if it means revisiting some of your "bottom lines."

Activity: Considering Common Challenge Areas

Here, we have identified a few areas that often pose challenges for parents of self-injuring youth. Included in each section are examples of common questions that tend to arise and a few issues to consider in your own personal deliberations and conversations. Before talking with your child about these issues, we encourage parents to first re-view these challenge areas and have a conversation with one another (if in a two-parent or co-parenting situation). Then, once common ground is reached, you will be better prepared to talk with your child.

For each of these identified challenge areas, consider the following:

1. What priority do you assign this particular area, and thus how critical is this as a focus for conversation and agreement?
2. What is and is not negotiable for you related to this general area?
3. What particular questions come up for you and/or other family members in this area?

We hope that this process will help you decide where to start the discussion and enable you to be very honest with your child about the strength of your feelings.

Key Challenges

WOUND DISPLAY

It can be difficult to see fresh wounds or even clustered scars. Frank conversation about everyone's desires and/or needs in this regard is useful, but it behooves parents to consider what is and is not negotiable before having this conversation. Consider the sensitivities and needs of everyone in the house. Primary questions here include: When and under what circumstances can fresh wounds be displayed? When and under what circumstances can old wounds or scars be displayed? Are the rules to be the same at home as while out in public together? At family outings or reunions?

- What specific questions/discussion points come to mind for you here?

- On a scale of 1 (not important) to 5 (very important), how critical is this issue as a focus for conversation and agreement?

- What is and is not negotiable for with regard to wound display?

WHAT TO TELL SIBLINGS

This is a challenging and common question for families with other kids in the house. The answer will largely depend on your family. Here are a few questions that typically come up: What do we tell siblings who have noticed something is going on, but who do not know any details? What do we tell siblings who know some details and who are clearly confused or worried? What do we tell siblings who know nothing at all? How do we help siblings not worry too much about their self-injuring brother or sister? What kind of support do they need as the family goes through this?

- What specific questions/discussion points come to mind for you here?

- On a scale of 1 (not important) to 5 (very important), how critical is this issue as a focus for conversation and agreement?

- What is and is not negotiable for you with regard to sharing information with siblings?

SHARING WITH EXTENDED FAMILY MEMBERS AND/OR CLOSE FRIENDS OF THE FAMILY

Extended family members or close family friends can be impacted as well, and many of the questions that come up for siblings can emerge for extended family members, particularly those who live close by and/or who are in regular contact with the family.

- What specific questions/discussion points come to mind for you here?

- On a scale of 1 (not important) to 5 (very important), how critical is this issue as a focus for conversation and agreement?

- What is and is not negotiable for you with regard to sharing information with extended family/close friends?

ENGAGEMENT IN FAMILY AND OTHER ACTIVITIES

Self-injury often comes along with depression, anxiety, or other conditions that result in youth pulling away from their families and social opportunities. Because of this, conversations and agreement about staying engaged in home and social activities are often necessary. Common questions that come up include: What is a reasonable level of engagement in activity at home, such as family dinners and outings? What is a reasonable level of engagement in structured activities outside of home (e.g., clubs, sports, social groups, or other extracurricular activities)? How do we negotiate relationships, friends, and activities that parents worry may be "triggers" for self-injury or unhealthy for their child?

- What specific questions/discussion points come to mind for you here?

- On a scale of 1 (not important) to 5 (very important), how critical is this issue as a focus for conversation and agreement?

- What is and is not negotiable for you with regard to engaging with family and other social opportunities?

PRIVACY

Issues related to privacy are among the first to arise for many parents. Restricting privacy, in particular, can cause any number of power struggles. Acknowledge any fears or worries you may have and give some thought to your non-negotiables and the points on which agreement may be possible—before power struggles happen. It may help to read the upcoming "Safety Concerns" section as you consider the kinds of issues likely to come up. Common questions include: How much privacy should my child have? What do we do about the possibility of self-injury happening at home? How much latitude should he or she have over decisions about whether or not to join family activities? How much alone time is too much? Take a minute to think about the types of questions you have related to privacy and, with these in mind, answer the questions below.

- What specific questions/discussion points come to mind for you here?

- On a scale of 1 (not important) to 5 (very important), how critical is this issue as a focus for conversation and agreement?

- What is and is not negotiable for you with regard to privacy issues?

ENGAGEMENT IN THERAPY

This is an area rife with very different expectations and experiences within families. There are many issues that come up for families around therapy, but the one that causes the most strife and that is worth discussion is expectations about attending therapy. Self-injury is often a tough thing to treat, and it is not uncommon for people who self-injure to dislike therapy or a therapist because they feel too pushed or not well understood. Because of this, going in and out of therapy or going for a while and then refusing to go again is not uncommon. This can cause a lot of friction in families since parents often think of therapy as a beacon of hope. Candid discussion of expectations about participation in therapy and how to find a therapist your child can work with often emerge as critical areas of discussion and agreement for families.

- What specific questions/discussion points come to mind for you here?

- On a scale of 1 (not important) to 5 (very important), how critical is this issue as a focus for conversation and agreement?

- What is and is not negotiable for you with regard to engaging in therapy?

RULES OF ENGAGEMENT AROUND EMOTIONAL TOPICS

This may be one of the most important subjects to talk about early on since negotiation in other areas may depend on the rules of engagement here. For example, what happens when one of you doesn't want to have a conversation? Are there times of the day or night that should be considered off-limits? How can you quickly let each other know that now is not a good time to talk about something hard or that one of you is having a bad day and could use a little extra space? Calmly coming up with agreed upon strategies for managing the "process of processing" can be helpful. Choosing cues, phrases, or other ways of quickly signaling "I am not open to talking," "not now but soon," or even "I need a hug but do not want to talk about it" can make some of the more difficult conversations and negotiations easier.

- What specific questions/discussion points come to mind for you here?

- On a scale of 1 (not important) to 5 (very important), how critical is this issue as a focus for conversation and agreement?

- What is and is not negotiable for you with regard to engaging in emotional conversations?

Safety Concerns

As a parent, your instinct is to do whatever you can to protect your child from harm. Physical harm—even self-inflicted—is something parents are hardwired to prevent. This means parents sometimes jump to extremes, such as taking doors off hinges to reduce privacy; removing all knives, scissors, and razor blades from the house so that there are no implements to injure with; or never leaving a child alone. While all of these impulses are understandable, it is wise to pause for a moment and reflect not only on the practicality of making these changes, but on whether or not they are helpful for your child.

For many who engage in the behavior, self-injury is about *control*. People who self-injure often see the behavior as the quickest and easiest route to self-soothing in moments of emotional distress or turmoil. Taking away all privacy or access to normal household items may actually *increase* this out-of-control feeling rather than make it better.

It is also important to consider your deeper intentions. Give yourself permission to experience feelings of sadness, frustration, or anger—but if you truly want to be an ally for your child, think about how to best show this in a way that is helpful to you

> Give yourself permission to experience feelings of sadness, frustration, or anger—but if you truly want to be an ally for your child, think about how to best show this in a way that is helpful to you both.

both. Keep in mind that a major aspect of changing self-injury behavior is being able to live and function in normal environments. Most normal household environments include scissors, knives, and so on. Even if you are able to temporarily remove all potential threats, your child will eventually need to learn to be and live in environments that include these things. (Moreover, know that people desperate to self-injure do not need specific tools or places to engage in the behavior—a variety of things you would not think to remove, like staples from magazines and things you cannot remove, like fingernails, can be used to self-injure. When really desperate to self-injure, a person will do it anywhere, even if this means others can see him do it.)

This being said, our recommendation is that you use your desire to limit your child's access to self-injury opportunities and tools as the starting point for conversation. Honestly share your feelings with your child and talk about why you feel the need to limit access to self-injury. Asking your child to also share his or her perceptions on safety concerns will likely provide you with insights and even some surprises. Some young people trying to change self-injury behavior find that some limitations are useful; for instance, having a go-to person who helps restrict the ability to act on self-injurious urges might give your child enough time to consider and try alternative coping methods in moments of distress. Other young people may resent the suggestion that you could or should control this aspect of their lives. In either case, when discussed at the right time (that is, when you are both calm and have the time for a conversation), this subject can offer an opportunity to agree on limits that you are both comfortable with, allowing you to work together to identify supports that would be useful *to both of you* during the change process.

Since individuals who injure may be emotionally volatile and may act out toward others, such as siblings or parents, in ways that inspire concern for personal well-being or safety, there must be clear agreements and consequences regarding aggressive behavior. Finding mindful and respectful strategies for diffusing tense moments can be particularly challenging in these cases (see the "Dealing with Power Struggles" section in the previous chapter). If aggression is an issue in your family, please be sure to enlist the help of your and your child's therapists in addressing it since aggression can be tremendously stressful for everyone.

The Pros and Cons of No-Harm Contracts

Parents may consider requiring a child to sign a "no-harm contract" (or enter into a similar verbal agreement), in which the child promises he or she will not self-injure. These contracts can also be between a patient and doctor. They can be formal contracts with signatures of all involved, or they can be informal, verbal agreements. Standard features of these contracts are an explicit statement saying that the individual will not harm or kill himself, specifics on the length of time the contract covers, a contingency plan if a crisis occurs, and the specific responsibilities of both/all parties. While some clinicians working with self-injurious clients use these contracts regularly in therapy, others believe they are not helpful. Youth who self-injure also have mixed responses to the idea. Some of the benefits and limitations of no-harm contracts are that they:

- convey a sense of responsibility and agency that underscores the seriousness of the issue and may increase the commitment level, active involvement, and sense of responsibility for oneself;
- provide structure and motivation for managing impulses that may become slips; and
- help parents and others who care feel like they are allies in the healing process.

For example, one self-injurious youth we spoke with said it was useful for him to know that his father was going to ask if he had self-injured on a weekly basis. This ongoing accountability to his father helped him in times of distress to remain focused on the longer term goal of quitting self-injury.

The limitations of no-harm contracts include:

- possibly becoming a symbolic power struggle when a youth perceives himself as being coerced;
- inadvertently shifting the focus away from gaining the skills needed to stop self-injury in the first place, overly focusing instead on the self-injury behavior;
- possibly setting the person who self-injures up to fail since it may not be possible to totally stop injuring right away, even with the best of intentions.

For instance, one youth reported feeling coerced into signing a no-harm contract by his therapist and parents and described intense feelings of shame and guilt when he had a self-injury slip, which led him to further hide his self-injury from his care providers.

An Alternative: Commitment to Treatment Statements

To move beyond these limitations, psychologists David Rudd and Thomas Joiner recommend use of what they refer to as a Commitment to Treatment Statement.[2] The treatment statement avoids use of the term "contract" and its legally binding connotations and instead emphasizes an agreement as an intervention that is part of a broader discussion and plan for moving forward. Here's an example of what this might look like, but this can be modified to suit your child's needs[2,3]:

I, _____, agree to make a commitment to taking care of myself. I understand that this means that I have agreed to be actively involved in:

(1) attending therapy sessions (or letting my therapist know when I can't make it),

(2) setting goals for myself,

(3) voicing my opinions, thoughts, and feelings honestly and openly with my parents and therapist (whether they are negative or positive, but most importantly my negative feelings),

(4) being actively involved in family outings and school commitments,

(5) completing homework assignments,

(6) experimenting with new healthy behaviors and new ways of doings things,

(7) and reaching out for help and implementing my crisis response plan when needed.

I also understand and acknowledge that, to a large degree, my healing depends on the amount of energy and effort I make. If I feel like something is not working at home, or treatment with my therapist is not working, I agree to discuss it with my therapist and attempt to come to a common understanding as to what the problems are and identify potential solutions. In short, I agree to make a commitment to living and treating my body well. This agreement will apply for the next three months, at which time it will be reviewed and modified.

Signed: _____

Date: _____

Regardless of whether you and your child decide that establishing a Commitment to Treatment Statement is right for both of you, we believe that the idea of it provides yet another opportunity for conversation with your child. Share your feelings, thoughts, and desires about a Commitment to Treatment Statement and ask your child about whether or not this kind of accountability would be useful. What are her thoughts, needs, and preferences? Would she prefer to have a statement such as this in writing, or does the prospect of a "formal" written statement cause anxiety? If your views on this differ widely, seek to reach a compromise and set a date to revisit the agreement. Always keep the door open for further dialogue about how to best support your child's goals related to self-injury.

Social Media and Self-Injury: What to Watch For

Use of the Internet and other social media platforms is nearly ubiquitous among young people. Nearly all adolescents and young adults access Internet-based applications, and many do so several times every day. Like everything else, self-injury–related content is very common across many different types of websites and social media platforms.

Popular apps tend to come and go, but the basics they allow users are relatively consistent. People who build or research the various features of websites and mobile applications describe these features in terms of "social affordances"—the ways in which people using social media are able to interact. For example, many currently popular apps, like Twitter, Instagram, and Snapchat, allow users to hide their identities with a username and/or image (often called an "avatar"). This allows users anonymity and can reduce barriers to sharing that might be present if the user were identifiable. Many platforms enable users to post images and videos, something very appealing to teens and young adults. Some apps have "geo" features that allow other users to see where the poster is located (usually a town rather than a street address is identifiable).

Posting and viewing self-injury–related material in social media is common. It is exceedingly easy to find self-injury communities and message boards, imagery, and videos. What happens in self-injury communities or in the social exchange occurring related to video posts (such as in the commentary section under YouTube videos) is widely variable. In some cases, posters and visitors gather to express feelings, exercise creative expression, solicit or give helpful support, or simply reassure each other that they are not alone. In other cases, the content and posts can be very triggering, can encourage negative behavior, and/or can lead to worsening self-injury behaviors or practices.

> It is exceedingly easy to find self-injury communities and message boards, imagery, and videos. What happens in self-injury communities or in the social exchange occurring related to video posts is widely variable.

While some may like to watch videos on sites like YouTube, others prefer online message boards like Tumblr where one can post images, text, and even video. Videos posted tend to be graphic, symbolic, or inspirational. One of the primary concerns regarding self-injury videos posted on Tumblr and YouTube is that the videos are often uploaded without trigger warnings and therefore are readily accessible to those who self-injure. Videos, images, and sound are powerful—often more powerful than words.

Research into self-injury and social media shows that most people who participate in online communities of individuals who self-injure believe that these communities support the healing process and encourage greater self-acceptance. Benefits of online exchange are especially strong for those who are very uncomfortable talking about self-injury offline or who have yet to disclose to anyone in their offline life. Depending on the nature of the exchange, what is shared can motivate introspection and increase the likelihood of taking proactive and productive steps to healing by allowing participants to bond over their experiences, console each other over relapses, and help each other on the healing path.[3]

This is why awareness is critical, but it is equally important to understand that effects of social media are not black and white. Use of social media and the Internet in general can be helpful or harmful or both depending on what and how it is used. On the more negative side, research has shown that exposure to self-injury images, videos, descriptions, or even reasons for self-injury can be very triggering for viewers, even if that is not the poster's intent. As Manuela describes:

> My self-injury definitely worsened after the Internet came along. There were so many chat rooms for people who self-injured. It did help in the short term but not in the long term. I have to avoid online self-injury communities now because they are so triggering.
> —*Manuela, on the contribution of social media to her self-injury*
> *(age 20)*

Many of the negative effects of online self-injury content are driven by its presentation. If the content does not emphasize positive behavior change or if it explicitly discourages ending self-injury, portrays self-injury as an effective and acceptable way of coping and a routine part of life (normalization), or as something aesthetically beautiful (glamorization), then it may encourage the behavior rather than support the individual in addressing the root of the behavior. Often, glamorization comes from the music and pictures in videos, which are sometimes appealing to viewers. Self-injury–focused content or communities may be especially harmful to viewers with no or limited experience with self-injury, as they show how it can be used as a coping mechanism, especially in a stressful situation. Being able to quickly find self-injury information or communities online may reduce motivation to seek more formal help and may reinforce the behavior. In general, social media that minimizes the effects, glamorizes, or normalizes self-injury can interfere with positive change.

Many web platforms have explicit guidelines prohibiting endorsement of self-injury. For example, while YouTube does not explicitly identify self-injury, it prohibits content which is dangerous or could cause injury. Tumblr explicitly indicates that content which leads to the "promotion or glorification of self-harm" is prohibited. Similarly, Instagram's policy guidelines do not allow posting of any content that glorifies self-injury, stating that any pictures that support self-injury will be taken down and offending user accounts disabled. Similarly, Twitter's policy guidelines include prohibition of "self-harm" related hashtags or tweets and explicitly warn users that mentions of self-injury or suicidality will be flagged and followed up by Twitter administrators. Facebook does not explicitly mention self-injury in its policy guidelines. It does, however, prohibit posts that encourage violence. Although formal policies do help in articulating and establishing community norms related to self-injury, there are a number of ways to circumvent the policy in any given forum. As a result, self-injury–related content remains quite common in every social media platform.

Even if youth are not participating in self-injury–specific forums, online and social media experiences can serve as both triggers and as buffers for the negative emotions and cognitions that often lead to the behavior. Applying respectful curiosity and deep listening skills to asking and understanding your child's online experience will be helpful in aiding your assessment of the role social media and other online activity may be playing relative to the self-injury behavior. You can also use your understanding to help your child come into deeper awareness of his or her patterns, since greater awareness brings a greater degree of choice. To assess the impact of this involvement on your child, you can ask questions such as:

- Where do you go most?
- What prompts you to go online? Have you noticed that experiencing certain emotions or thoughts may lead you there more quickly?
- How do you feel after you go online to talk with others about self-injury?
- What do you think the effect has been on your healing process?
- Have you ever seen or read anything that triggered you? If so, how did you handle it?
- Do you ever worry about how you feel when you go online or what you see or do there?

Social media and other virtual forums are a standard part of twenty-first-century life for young people and adults. Advances in new technology will expand the way all of us interact with others in ways that most of us cannot even fathom right now. Helping youth foster online presences and exchanges that are fundamentally supportive of them and others is a parent's best long-term strategy. It is not always easy to know exactly what your child is doing with regard to social media, particularly if he or she is older. Helping young people ask and answer the following questions can be helpful:

- Are the places and communities you visit helping or hindering your goal of not self-injuring anymore?
- How much time do you spend online in general and related to self-injury in particular? (A lot of time spent in online forums, even if your child perceives that they are supportive, is likely to interfere with healing since so much of the skills they need to acquire relate to meaningful and satisfying engagement in offline life.)

Note that instead of banning sites, directing youth toward healthier and more beneficial avenues of self-injury expression over social media is a more effective strategy to help. Focus also on enhancing "Internet literacy" skills whenever possible. Media education can start at home, with parents educating their children about recognizing media messages and questioning the underlying ideas and beliefs expressed. Watching popular but potentially triggering shows together can provide opportunities for revealing and useful exchanges of perspectives. In addition, there are a number of useful online media literacy resources for this, such as Common Sense Media (commonsensemedia.org/social-media), the Center for Media Literacy (medialit.net), and Safe Smart Social (safesmartsocial.com).

Collaborations Critical
for Ending Self-Injury

I would encourage them to not go it alone. To seek a compassionate person, whether it be a psychologist or friend . . . to make sure you let your emotions be known. To not hold it all in. To share and let people share with you. And realize that in most cases this is not something that you necessarily had control of and you really can't do anything about it because it is in your past, I mean, it's happened. So all you can do is work toward trying to make it better. And part of making it better is making yourself better. And not feeling that overwhelming guilt that comes with it. So, that's what I would say.

—Advice from a dad

Wanting to find help while simultaneously wanting to limit the number of people who know about a child's self-injury is a common dilemma for parents. The desire to find help for a child often takes precedence and generally results in finding a therapist (or turning to one already known to the family). As we have noted, despite the fact that parental self-care is vital, it is not terribly common for parents to look for therapeutic support for themselves during this time. Moreover, parents often face challenging decisions about who else to confide in and what exactly to tell them. This is because self-injury can be a very difficult thing to talk about, and not just because it a sensitive topic. Should some family or friends be told while others are left in the dark? Should a child's school be involved? If so, who specifically should parents talk to? What should be shared, and what should be held back? How might sharing affect the receiver's perception of one's family, child, or oneself? It can be so confusing and contain so many unknowns that it is not at all surprising that some people choose to tell no one at all.

While we do know that confiding in people can be very hard, especially if they are not already close to the family in some way, we do suggest that you identify potential allies and collaborators in supporting your child's healing and your own well-being. Because we understand how tough it can be to navigate all of these decisions and feelings, this chapter is devoted to ensuring that you have the support you need to support your child. We cannot tell you exactly who to talk to or exactly what to say, but we can offer some guidance.

Key People and Institutions: The Perspectives They Bring and How They Can Help

In putting together a support network, it can be helpful to think broadly about key resources and what they each offer. Support comes in many forms: emotional support, instrumental (or tactical) support, and/or resource bridges. *Emotional supporters* often listen, empathize, reflect, and/or encourage. *Instrumental supporters* help with the daily or periodic details of everyday life in tangible ways, such as driving to/from appointments, helping with running errands, and the like. *Resource bridges* are supports that help link you to other needed resources, such as people (e.g., therapist recommendations) or things (e.g., financial assistance, "how-to" supports). Knowing whether you are asking for support for you, your child, or your family (or specific members of your family, such as siblings who are affected) is helpful. In all likelihood, you will

> Think carefully about how to recruit a network of support that covers all members of your family.

want to think carefully about how to recruit a network of support that covers all members of your family.

Deciding When, How, What, and with Whom to Share

There are a few things to consider in deciding when, how, and with whom to share. While allowing for authentic exchange is an important part of the process, spending a little time to think about your motives and goals for sharing can help bring into better focus the *what* to share. It can also help you articulate what you hope to get out of the relationship and who to share with, when, and how. Each of these is discussed here, with space for you write down your thoughts.

Why Share?

It is useful to think a little about why you want to tell someone your child is self-injuring. Here are some common questions to consider: What are you seeking? Do you want emotional support? A friendly ear for the hard times and/or someone to celebrate the small successes? Or, do you need logistical or tactical support—someone who can help with transportation or kid care or figuring out how to keep life going when your attention may be pulled in too many directions? Perhaps you need financial assistance or help in identifying local therapeutic resources? Whatever it is, it is helpful to be as clear as possible with yourself so that you can ask for, and hopefully receive, what you need.

Consider here why you want to share, and what you want to get out of sharing:

Confiding simply because you feel like you *should* share makes sense with a spouse or your child's other parent(s) or possibly with siblings, but it is still helpful to think about what you might hope to accomplish with this sharing. Simply recruiting allies for your child or to help you is enough, but there may well be other reasons to share. Remember that obtaining support for yourself *is* a way of supporting your child. You matter a lot, so anything that supports and stabilizes you will help your child and your family. Once you know why you want to share, it is helpful to let that person know why you chose to share this information with him or her. Starting the conversation with something candid, such as, "I just need someone to listen right now," or "I could really use some advice," can help prepare the listener for the seriousness of the topic.

What to Share?

While it can feel very cathartic to share the "whole story," it can also make one feel very vulnerable, or it can feel otherwise unhelpful. You do not need to share everything, all the vivid details, events, associated thoughts and feelings, to effectively solicit support. If sharing that your child is self-injuring feels too exposing, then consider stating simply that your child is struggling right now and that it has been difficult for everyone in the family. Sometimes sharing the specifics can distract from the main point of the conversation, depending on what you decide about your reasons for *why* you're sharing in the first place. If you do share some specifics of the self-injury, be prepared for the possibility that you will need to educate your confidante about it—many people do not know what it is or understand that it is not a suicide attempt.

What information would be useful to share about your situation? What do you think you should avoid sharing?

Who to Reach Out To?

Next, you'll want to identify those people in the best position to help and who are likely to be able to hear what you have to share without judgment. Even in cases where someone does not need to know much to provide you with information, resources, or support, you will need to provide some context, so approaching someone you trust is important.

Who are the people that you think you can trust to understand you and withhold judgment? If you have shared confidential information with him or her in the past, did you feel supported afterward? Was there any reason you wish you had not shared, or wished that you had shared less detail? Was he or she able to keep your conversation private?

Keep in mind that you do not need many confidantes to feel supported—even one can make a big difference in your sense of well-being. Not everyone you know is a good candidate for supporting you during this time, but it is likely that some are. Also, keep in mind that if the other person is also currently dealing with difficult issues, he or she might not be able to provide you with the support you seek. Use the space provided below to answer the questions above.

When, Where, and How to Have That First Conversation?

It helps to think a little about when and where to have the first conversation with someone you want to confide in. This is something you will want to discuss privately. Face-to-face conversation is often the most comfortable, but if that is too hard or if the person you want to talk to does not live nearby, a phone conversation may work just as well. Just be sure that you have set aside enough time for you to say all that you want to say, as well as for the other person to ask questions, without interruptions or distractions. You will also want to make sure that both of you are calm when you share this information as it is likely to evoke emotion. Keep in mind you can always put off the conversation and come back to it at another, better time. If the conversation becomes uncomfortable for any reason, you do not have to continue. Having educational materials or resources on hand can also be helpful since it is common for individuals to have a number of questions that may be easily answered with such materials.

What thoughts do you have about when, where, and how you plan to share?

Talking to Your Child's Friends

Your child's friends may well be the first to know or suspect that your son or daughter is self-injuring. It may even be through a friend that you first find out about the self-injury or that you turn to in order to learn more detail. This is very understandable, and friends can be strong and important allies. That said, it is important to be mindful of not putting your child's friends in awkward or untenable positions by demanding information from them. They are likely to be walking a very fine line between maintaining your child's (their

> It is important to be mindful of not putting your child's friends in awkward or untenable positions by demanding information from them.

friend's) confidence and helping you stay informed. They may feel like they are risking an important relationship and may be understandably conflicted about what to share. It can be very helpful to let them know, for example, that you do not want to put them in a compromising position and that you do not want them to report on or "tell on" their friend, your child. The easiest to honor agreement will be one in which you both agree that he or she will let you know if they notice anything that worries them more than usual and/or if something changes that may signal a turn for the worse. Asking them to let you know if they are noticing positive change, as well, can give them an opportunity to share good news with you and not just the hard stuff.

What to Do when Your Child's Friends May Be Part of the Problem

Your child's friends can be powerful allies in helping him or her to change self-injury behavior. Indeed, friendships are a necessary and generally healthy part of life; but it is also true that some friendships can be harmful and destructive. When an unhealthy or destructive behavior such as self-injury spreads among a group of friends or peers, this can be a form of social contagion. Parents should be aware that social contagion can become an issue among members of a group of friends or peers. This is particularly common in schools, but can occur in any social setting and involve a small group of friends or a large outbreak across multiple school grades.

Social contagion is a risk any time others become aware that someone among them is injuring. Dr. Barent Walsh notes in his book for mental health professionals, *Treating Self-Injury: A Practical Guide,* that certain behaviors are susceptible to social contagion both because of their power to communicate as well as the provocative nature of the act itself. The risk for contagion is increased when high-status or "popular" peers are engaged in self-injury or when self-injury is used as a means for students to feel a sense of cohesiveness or belonging to a particular group. The point here is not to figure out "who started it," but to stop the behavior from occurring and spreading further. In a school setting, this is most typically done by reducing the group's communication about self-injury. If a student is injuring, for example, he or she should be advised not to explicitly talk with other students about engaging in the behavior and be instructed to cover visible scars and wounds. If a broader conversation in the group does occur, the focus should be on helping to come up with ideas for using positive coping skills.

How can you help your child negotiate relationships with friends who you worry may be "triggering" for self-injury or who are otherwise unhealthy for your child? This is a time to put to use the skills that you have learned in the past few chapters. Begin by openly and genuinely sharing your concerns with your child about the relationship he has with the friend(s) you have concerns about. The aim is to have a candid conversation about the nature of this friendship and its pros and cons. For instance, consider the difference between these two statements: "I don't ever want you to hang out with Alexa again," versus "I would like to reserve the right to not have you spend time with Alexa when I feel like you are in a vulnerable space, okay?" Imagine how your child might react to each of these statements. How might *you* react if you were in his shoes? Which of these statements allows for conversation and keeping the proverbial "communication door" open? If you are open to having your child challenge this and to sharing what you observe, you may both arrive at a deeper understanding of each other and yourselves. You may also arrive at an *agreement* rather than a *mandate,* and this seemingly small difference can have very powerful consequences. As we discussed in previous chapters, rarely do positive steps come from laying down the law with hard and fast rules for your child. No one wants to be told who they can or can't see or be friends with. The intent of an open and constructive conversation is to come to a mutually acceptable agreement that allows you and your child to gain a deeper understanding of the various perspectives involved.

> No one wants to be told who they can or can't see or be friends with.

Institutions

In addition to tapping individuals in your informal network for support, it can be useful to think about how to best work with the institutions or groups with which your child spends significant time. Schools are the most common institution in this category, but not the only one. Any group your child is a part of, such as an athletic team or art/theater group, may be a source of important and useful allies. Much of this depends, of course, on the extent to which your child's mental health challenges are known by the group leaders. There is no reason to raise alarm or to complicate your child's life by assuming that everyone she has contact with knows everything. Connecting with the individuals who may have shared concerns, who are natural allies because of the amount of time they spend with your child, or because they are likely to be well-equipped to assist in some way can extend the cloak of protection you want for your child.

Working with Schools

School professionals such as teachers, nurses, and counselors are frequently some of the first adults to know or suspect a student's self-injury. Athletic coaches or adults affiliated with school groups your child is a part of may also be among the first to notice mood changes or actual wounds or scars, especially in sports where shorts, bathing suits, or short-sleeve shirts may be required. In some cases, students self-disclose that they are self-injuring. In other cases, a peer might notify a staff member of another student's self-injury. In still other cases, a teacher, counselor, or staff member might first notice signs suggesting that a student is self-injuring, such as repeated instances of injuries or bandages or wearing long sleeves during warm weather. School staff will hopefully be trained to recognize that self-injury is not limited to a particular look or appearance nor is it confined to membership in a particular social group.

Ongoing Collaborative Relationships with the School

In an ideal world, school staff, in particular the school's point person, would be able to collaborate with the student, family members, and any involved mental health providers to ensure that the student gets the assistance and support she needs. Ideally this would involve sustained relationships of mutual respect and collaboration and positive and open communications. While schools will not likely play a role in any formal therapy for the student or her family, they will want to ensure that each of their students is able to learn and grow in the academic environment. For instance, for some students, school-based psychologists or other mental health staff may be able to assist with counseling for the issues underlying the self-injury. For other students, referral to other external supports, such as individual or family therapy, may be warranted. Having a conversation with the school's point person about what the school is able to offer your child and what your child needs will be helpful in going forward so that you are all on the same page.

Typical School Protocols

The protocol a school follows when staff become aware of self-injury varies by school and district but there are often consistencies. When a staff member notices that a student has wounds, suspects that a student is injuring, or has the behavior brought to his or her attention by another student, it is common for a designated point person, usually a school nurse or counselor, to be alerted. That person might engage with the student first to assess the extent and nature of the self-injury. Whether the school will engage the student as a collaborator in deciding a course of action once self-injury is disclosed (such as deciding who is going to tell you—the student or the school) really varies from school to school. We, like many of our colleagues, recommend that schools do provide the student as many choices as possible within their protocol guidelines. For example, it may be required that the school notify you, the parent, but the school can provide the student with the choice of calling you herself or letting the designated point person make the call. Your child benefits from knowing that she has a say in how she is treated at school. The school is likely to need to know about self-injury severity and chronicity and to want to be sure that your child and/or family is receiving outside support. They may also need to ask questions about your child's history and/or experience in the home just to be confident that your child is well supported. Since the presence of self-injury can spark concerns about abuse, the school is likely to err on the side of caution here. Since self-injury can also be a risk factor for suicidal thoughts and behaviors, as you know, the school is likely to need to periodically assess suicidal thoughts and behaviors as well.

> Since self-injury can also be a risk factor for suicidal thoughts and behaviors, as you know, the school is likely to need to periodically assess suicidal thoughts and behaviors as well.

If suicidality is detected, suicide protocols will be followed, meaning that your child would likely be transferred to the hospital for professional assessment and treatment.

What Is a Parent's Role?

In many districts, a meeting between the student, parents, and the point person or crisis team will be scheduled soon after the self-injury is detected or disclosed. The meeting is likely to cover the following issues:

- *Basic education.* The point person who speaks with you will fill you in on what the school knows and how they know it. If you lack information about self-injury, they will likely do some basic education (at least they should) or provide you with resources that will contain the information you need.
- *Provision of resources.* One of the most important mandates the school will face is assuring that you know that self-injury is generally best treated by a professional therapist and then assuring that you are linked to external community-based resources. They may also speak with you about the value of family therapy and may offer to assist with setting up initial appointments. They may also periodically check in with you about how therapy is going for your child and/or to be sure you have other supports in place.
- *Create and maintain a supportive environment.* Ideally, the school point person or team will work with parents and the student to figure out how to create and maintain a supportive, appropriate environment. These conversations may include assuring academic support, assessing the social support resources and needs of your child, and helping to find strategies for dealing with external challenges such as financial barriers or unexpected challenges or setbacks. It may also be useful for the school crisis team and/or point person to be able to communicate with any outside professionals who are assisting your child. In this case, you may be asked to authorize release of information to the schools and professionals.
- *Follow-up meetings.* Ideally, you can see the school as part of your child's caring team. Making sure you know who is most knowledgeable about your child's case and staying in touch about her life at school can help you feel supported as well as

ensure that everyone has the most up-to-date information. It is not necessary to share all details, of course, but it helps if you can agree on the general state of progress and areas where your child would benefit from additional support. It is also quite uplifting to share successes. The school may want to schedule follow-up meetings as well. These typically occur 1–2 weeks and no later than 1 month after the school detects a self-injury incident. A follow-up meeting offers a good opportunity for checking in to see what obstacles the family has encountered and what additional resources the school may be able to help with facilitating. Remember that school professionals are available to help with sorting out what needs to be done to help their students flourish.

What Are the Legal Issues Surrounding Parent Notification and Self-Injury?

The American School Counselor Association requires confidentiality between students and counselors *except* in the event that the student is at risk for harm. Because self-injury is so often a coping behavior and not an actual attempt to die (e.g., suicide), experts in self-injury generally recommend that elementary and secondary school staff inform parents about their child's self-injuring behavior even in cases where it is likely or clear that the child is not an immediate threat to himself or herself. It is important for parents to know that the school also has a responsibility to assure that they release the child to adequate parental care. In cases where a parent is clearly disengaged or not willing to set up outside assistance, the school may determine that the parents are being neglectful. Because schools are mandated reporters, the school does have the responsibility to report parental neglect to the local child protection agency.

Mental Health Providers as Allies

It is very likely that your child will see a therapist at some point in the healing process. She may even see multiple individuals over time since it can be challenging in some cases to find a good "fit." As we discussed in Chapter 6, if there are multiple diagnoses and concerning behaviors, such as suicide attempts, your child may benefit from residing in a therapeutic care center for a short while. No matter what the therapeutic environment is, however, it is important for you to know that therapists are bound by confidentiality rules that may limit what they can share with you about your child's process. While this can sometimes be frustrating, it is useful to know that your child's therapist is an ally.

Activity

How Do You Feel?

You answered these questions early on in this book. Take a few moments to consider them once more, in light of everything you know now and everything you've done in the course of reading this book.

1. On a scale of 1–7 where 1 = Very comfortable, 7 = Very uncomfortable, and N/A = not applicable, how comfortable do you currently feel:

    a) Talking to your child about his/her/their self-injury _____
    b) Sharing your hopes, fears, and feelings with at least one other family member _____
    c) Talking with your child's siblings about your child's self-injury _____
    d) Sharing your hopes, fears, and other feelings with at least one other person outside your immediate family (such as a friend) _____
    e) Finding support resources, such as therapy, for your child _____
    f) Seeking or participating in therapy for yourself (e.g., individuals rather than family therapy) _____
    g) Talking about your child's challenges and needs with other adults in your child's life who may be helpful such as school, therapist, or group/ program leaders _____

2. How confident are you about the following issues:

Scale: Goes from 1–7 with 1 = Very confident and 7 = Not at all confident

    a) My child will eventually stop self-injuring _____
    b) My child will eventually thrive _____
    c) My child will be stronger as a result of these challenges _____
    d) I will be stronger as a result of these challenges _____

Take a look at the scores you gave to these questions at the end of the "Why This Book and Why Now" section on page 5. What has changed? Are you more or less optimistic, hopeful, and aware of resources?

Appendix

Tools and Resources

Nationally Recognized Self-Injury Treatment Programs

The Bridge of Central Massachusetts, offering inpatient and
  outpatient therapeutic services for adults, adolescents, and
  children: https://www.thebridgecm.org
SAFE ALTERNATIVES is a nationally recognized treatment
  approach, professional network, and educational resource base,
  which is committed to helping you and others achieve an end
  to self-injurious behavior: https://selfinjury.com/

Self-Injury Resources

The Cornell Research Program on Self-Injury and
  Recovery: www.selfinjury.bctr.cornell.edu/resources.html
Self-Injury Outreach and Support: www.sioutreach.org

Self-Injury Foundation: www.selfinjuryfoundation.org/
Inspiring Connections: www.inspiringconnections.ca/

Learning More About Your Parenting Style

A helpful website developed by Vanderbilt University
that describes the types of parenting styles and
how to identify yours: https://my.vanderbilt.
edu/developmentalpsychologyblog/2013/12/
types-of-parenting-styles-and-how-to-identify-yours/
Another useful description of the four main types of
parenting style and a brief critique of this literature
and its shortcomings: https://www.verywell.com/
parenting-styles-2795072

Resources on Treatment

Theravive, is a network of licensed and professional
counsellors, therapists, and psychologists who uphold
clear, compassionate values in therapy. Theravive's
purpose is to connect you to the right professional,
giving you a better direction, new goals, and a clearer
understanding of how to get there: https://www.
theravive.com/
Behavioral Tech, LLC, trains mental healthcare providers and
treatment teams who work with complex populations to use
compassionate, scientifically valid treatments and to implement
and evaluate these treatments in their practice setting. Their
website has a variety of helpful resources including a therapist
directory: http://behavioraltech.org/index.cfm
Talkspace.com is a digital therapy resource, allowing users to
engage with a therapist at any time on their smartphone or
through the web. It provides "affordable, confidential, and
anonymous therapy at the touch of a button." This can be a
great resource for parents who feel they do not have the time

for in-person therapy appointments or do not have many treatment resources available locally: www.talkspace.com

Mindfulness Resources

It's important to set a regular time to disconnect and unplug. It seems counterintuitive, doesn't it? There are some fantastic resources available online and apps that allow you to tune in, take a break, slow down, and connect with yourself—for as much time as your day allows. Most mindfulness practices require only yourself and a space to be in that helps you to feel calm and peaceful. Here are some mindfulness and meditation apps and websites that we've found helpful:

Stop, Breathe & Think. A free web and mobile app that opens with a short "interview" where users select several words to describe how they are feeling at that moment; then the app recommends guided meditations for mindfulness and compassion that are based on the user's current state. We've had several students use this app throughout the semester in order to tune in to themselves and work on reducing their stress levels, all with positive results: www. stopbreathethink.org

Smiling Mind. A free web and mobile mindfulness app, this not-for-profit group designed this program to provide "clarity, calm, and contentment": http://smilingmind.com.au

Take a Break! This app provides short, guided meditations for stress relief and much needed breaks during the day and can be listened to for either 7 or 13 minutes: https://itunes.apple.com/ us/app/take-break!-guided-meditations/id4.53857236?mt=8

Calm. Subscription website and free basic version available for iPhone with guided meditation and relaxation exercises. The guides and programs included cover topics such as body scans to help identify areas of stress, calming anxiety, getting deep sleep, emergency calm during stressful moments, and seven days of gratitude: https://www.calm.com

Insight Timer. A free mobile app with virtual "bells" to time and support your meditations, as well as various ambient sounds that can be played while you are tuning out and turning in. It's also pretty cool to see how many people around the world are meditating with you: https://insighttimer.com/timer

Headspace. Meditation made simple; this website and app are billed as "your gym membership for the mind." This app has a free 10-day introductory period of 10-minute mindfulness and meditation activities, after which it requires a paid subscription to continue to use. You can track your progress with stats and engage with friends, too: https://www.headspace.com

Other Helpful Websites

The Crisis Text Lineserves young people in any type of crisis, providing them access to free, 24/7 emotional support and information they need via the medium they already use and trust—texting: www.crisistextline.org/

National Suicide Prevention Lifeline. If you feel you are in a crisis, *whether or not* you are thinking about killing yourself, please call the Lifeline. People have called for help with substance abuse, economic worries, relationship and family problems, sexual orientation, illness, getting over abuse, depression, mental and physical illness, and even loneliness. By calling 1-800-273-TALK (8255), you'll be connected to a skilled, trained counselor at a crisis center in your area, *anytime 24/7*. There is also the feature to chat with someone from 2 PM until 2 AM, daily: www.suicidepreventionlifeline.org/

ChronicleMe (CMe) is a new social media site that will allow you to share details of your life that you may not want to share with 500 of your closest Facebook friends. Whether it is an embarrassing tidbit about yourself or a secret that you just are not ready to share with the world, CMe will serve as a one-stop shop for all your emotional needs. With its two distinct online communities, CMe Support and CMe Laugh, CMe will give users the freedom to share everyday thoughts anonymously while only receiving positive reinforcement from like-minded people who may be in the same situation. It's a judgment-free environment in which users control their anonymity by choosing if and when they reveal themselves to another user: www.cmelaugh.com/signup

Effective Child Therapy is an excellent resource for information on evidence-based treatments for children and adolescents struggling with mental health: http://effectivechildtherapy.org/

Psychwire.org is a new social media site for researchers, practitioners, and allied professionals of mental health and behavioral science. It is designed to provide opportunities for networking within a supportive forum of researchers and therapists. As an international project, it aims to encourage lively global dialogue and Q&A and to promote sharing of useful resources including research, books, documents, and media: www. psychwire.org.

Loveislouder.com provides support to those feeling mistreated or alone. The project is designed to engage individuals in expressing their feelings and promotes positive thinking, words, and behaviors in communities: www.loveislouder.com

Emotionsanonymous.org. The EA membership is composed of people who come together in weekly meetings for the purpose of working toward recovery from emotional difficulties. EA members are from many walks of life and are of diverse ages, economic status, and social and educational backgrounds. The only requirement for membership is a desire to become well emotionally: www.emotionsanonymous.org

GetSomeHeadspace. Headspace is a project designed to demystify meditation. Using the wonders of science and technology, they make it easy to learn, fun to do, and relevant to your everyday life. This is meditation for modern life—simple, scientifically proven techniques that you can use every day to experience a healthier and happier mind. The Headspace website goes into the science behind mindfulness and meditation and helps users learn how to use meditation skills to help overcome anxiety, depression, stress, addiction, and more: www. GetSomeHeadspace

ReachOut.com. This organization provides online resources for youth struggling with mental health issues. The site gives users the opportunity to build peer support networks through forums and presents extensive information through fact sheets, blogs, and other online tools. Find ReachOut.com's resources specifically on self injury at: http://us.reachout.com/facts/self-harm

Strengthofus.org is an online community providing resources on positive thinking to those struggling with mental health issues. Users can read blogs, participate in forums, or read and listen to the great content featured on the website: www.strengthofus.org

Critical Mental Health Resources for College Students. This website is meant to provide college students and young people with quality information on maintaining good mental health and identifying mental health issues: www.onlinecolleges.net/for-students/mental-health-resources

The American Academy of Child and Adolescent Psychiatry is aimed at helping parents and families in understanding emotional, developmental, behavioral, and mental disorders affecting children: www.aacap.org

The National Mental Health Association has an online factsheet about self-injury available at: www.nmha.org/index.cfm?objectid=C7DF982C-1372-4D20-C828323203058E6C

To Write Love on Her Arms is a nonprofit movement dedicated to presenting hope and finding help for people struggling with depression, addiction, self-injury, and suicide. TWLOHA exists to encourage, inform, inspire, and also to invest directly into treatment and recovery: http://twloha.com

Notes

Chapter 1

1. Whitlock, Purington, & Gershkovich, M. (2009).
2. Brumberg (2006).
3. See http://itriples.org/self-injury/
4. American Psychiatric Association (2013).
5. Learn more about the DSM-5 here: https://www.psychiatry.org/psychiatrists/practice/dsm.
6. Swannell, Martin, Page, Hasking, & St. John (2014).
7. See Whitlock & Selekman (2014) for review.
8. Swannell, Martin, Page, Hasking, & St. John (2014).
9. Martin, Swannell, Harrison, Hazell, & Taylor (2010).
10. Lloyd-Richardson, Perrine, Dierker, & Kelley (2007); Whitlock et al. (2011).
11. Whitlock et al. (2011).
12. Muehlenkamp, Hilt, Ehlinger, & McMillan (2015).
13. Whitlock et al. (2011).
14. Hawton, Rodham, Evans, & Weatherall, R. (2002).
15. Purington, Whitlock, Pochtar (unpublished ms).
16. Nock, Joiner, Gordon, Lloyd-Richardson, & Prinstein (2007).
17. Brown, Comtois, & Linehan (2002).
18. Nock, Joiner, Gordon, Lloyd-Richardson, & Prinstein (2007).
19. Ross, Heath, & Toste (2009).
20. Turner, Austin, & Chapman (2015).
21. Kleindienst et al. (2008).
22. Zetterqvist (2015).
23. Bresin & Schoenleber (2015)
24. Serras, Saules, Cranford, & Eisenberg (2010).
25. Walsh (2012).

26. Whitlock et al. (2013).
27. Klonsky (2011).
28. Whitlock et al. (2013).

Chapter 2

1. Kelada, Whitlock, Hasking, & Melvin (2016).
2. Marotz & Kupzyk (2018).
3. Baetens et al. (2014).
4. Yehuda & Bierer (2007).
5. McGowan et al. (2009); Weaver et al. (2004).
6. https://www.ted.com/talks/moshe_szyf_how_early_life_experience_is_written_into_dna/transcript?language=en
7. See https://www.nature.com/nature/journal/v531/n7592_supp/full/531S18a.html
8. Di Pierro et al. (2012).
9. Hilt, Nock, Lloyd-Richardson, & Prinstein (2008).
10. Whitlock, Lloyd-Richardson, Fisseha, & Bates (2017).

Chapter 3

1. Learn more about the DSM-V here: https://www.psychiatry.org/psychiatrists/practice/dsm
2. Merikangas et al. (2010).
3. Brumberg (1997); Lader (2006).
4. Whitlock, Purington, & Gershkovich (2009).
5. Steinberg & Morris (2001).
6. Favazza (1996).
7. PEW Research Foundation: http://www.pewresearch.org/
8. The American Freshman: National Norms Fall 2014. https://www.heri.ucla.edu/monographs/TheAmericanFreshman2014.pdf

Chapter 4

1. This quote was republished with permission from tinybuddha.com. You can find the original post here: https://tinybuddha.com/blog/when-painful-things-happen-and-you-dont-understand-why/
2. Glassman et al. (2007).
3. Brumariu & Kerns (2010).
4. Cox et al. (2012).
5. Arbuthnott & Lewis (2015).
6. Walsh (2012).
7. Ibid.
8. Hawton, Saunders, & O'Connor (2012).
9. Althoff et al. (2012).
10. Zeanah et al. (2005).
11. Maciejewski et al. (2014).
12. Sher & Stanley (2009).
13. Groschwitz & Plener (2012).

14. Ibid.
15. Wallenstein & Nock (2007).
16. Hyde, Conroy, Pincus, & Ram (2011).
17. Josefsson, Lindwall, & Archer (2014).
18. Stanton, Happell, Hayman, & Reaburn (2014).
19. McPhie & Rawana (2015).
20. Klonsky & Glenn (2008).
21. Thayer, Newman, & McClain (1994).
22. US Department of Health and Human Services (2008).
23. Gilbert (2012).
24. Franklin, Lee, Hanna, & Prinstein (2013).
25. Ibid.
26. Walsh (2012).
27. Chapman, Gratz, & Brown (2006).
28. Victor & Klonsky (2014b).
29. See https://selfinjury.com/
30. Nock & Mendes (2008).
31. Walsh (2012).
32. Lloyd-Richardson, Perrine, Dierker, & Kelley (2007).

Chapter 5

1. Whitlock, Prussein, & Pietrusza (2015).
2. Andresen et al. (2006).
3. Prochaska, DiClemente, & Norcross (1992).
4. Victor & Klonsky (2014a).
5. Kelada, Hasking, & Melvin (2016).
6. Kelada, Whitlock, Hasking, & Melvin (2016); Oldershaw, Richards, Simic, & Schmidt (2008); Byrne et al. (2008).

Chapter 6

1. Whitlock, Prussein, & Pietrusza (2015).
2. Fox et al. (2015).
3. Walsh (2012).
4. Muehlenkamp, Brausch, Quigley, & Whitlock (2012).
5. Nock et al. (2006).
6. Whitlock, Prussein, & Pietrusza (2015).
7. Pietrusza, Rothenberg, & Whitlock (2011, June).

Chapter 7

1. Walsh (2012).
2. Healthypsych (n.d.), https://healthypsych.com/family-therapy/; Hollander (2012).
3. Andover, Morris, Wren, & Bruzzese (2012).
4. Wedig & Nock (2007).
5. Glenn, Franklin, & Nock (2015).
6. Diamond et al. (2002).

7. Pineda & Dadds (2013).
8. Kendall et al. (2008).
9. Esposito-Smythers et al. (2011); Glenn, Franklin, & Nock (2015).
10. Esposito-Smythers et al. (2011).
11. Spirito, Esposito-Smythers, Wolff, & Uhl (2011).
12. Linehan (2014).
13. Linehan, Heard, & Armstrong (1993).
14. Rathus & Miller (2002); Fleischhaker et al. (2011).
15. Rathus & Miller (2002).
16. Andover, Schatten, Morris, & Miller (2015).
17. D'Zurilla & Nezu (2001); Muehlenkamp (2006).
18. Evans et al. (1999).
19. Tyrer et al. (2003).
20. Townsend et al. (2001).
21. Hollander (2008).
22. Plener, Libal, & Nixon (2009); Sandman (2009).
23. Harper (2012).
24. Nickel et al. (2006); Nickel, Loew, & Gil (2007).
25. Andresen, Oades, & Caputi (2003).

Chapter 8

1. Roepke & Seligman (2015).
2. Whitlock, Prussein, & Pietrusza (2015).
3. Whitlock, Lloyd-Richardson, Fisseha, & Bates (2017).
4. Dweck (2012).
5. Mangels et al. (2006).
6. Wood, Froh, & Geraghty (2010).

Chapter 9

1. Boas (2013).
2. Gilbert (1998).
3. Burns (1980).

Chapter 10

1. Kabat-Zinn (2003, p. 145).
2. Chiesa & Serretti (2010).
3. Linehan (1993).
4. Duncan, Coatsworth, & Greenberg (2009); also see Kabat-Zinn (2009).
5. Linehan (2014).
6. Open, honest questions come from a set of practices known as the Circle of Trust approach developed by the Center for Courage & Renewal and based on the work of author/educator Parker J. Palmer. Learn more at www.couragerenewal.org.
7. Garland et al. (2010).

Chapter 12

1. For NSSI resources developed specifically for parents, see http://www.selfinjury. bctr.cornell.edu/resources.html and http://sioutreach.org/learn-self-injury/

2. Taken from Jobes, Rudd, Overholser, & Joiner (2008, p. 405).

3. Marchant et al. (2017).

References

Althoff, R. R., Hudziak, J. J., Willemsen, G., Hudziak, V., Bartels, M., & Boomsma, D. I. (2012). Genetic and environmental contributions self-reported thoughts of self-harm and suicide. *American Journal of Medical Genetics B Neuropsychiatry and Genetics, 159B*(1), 120–127.

The American Freshman: National Norms Fall 2014. https://www.heri.ucla.edu/monographs/TheAmericanFreshman2014.pdf

American Psychiatric Association. (2013). *Diagnostic and statistical manual of mental disorders* (5th ed.). Arlington, VA: American Psychiatric Publishing.

Andover, M. S., Morris, B. W., Wren, A., & Bruzzese, M. E. (2012). Occurrence of non-suicidal self-injury and attempted suicide among adolescents: Distinguishing risk factors and psychosocial correlates. *Child & Adolescent Psychiatry & Mental Health, 6*(11), 1–7.

Andover, M. S., Schatten, H. T., Morris, B. W., & Miller, I. W. (2015). Development of an intervention for nonsuicidal self-injury in young adults: An open pilot trial. *Cognitive and Behavioral Practice, 22*(4), 491–503.

Andresen, R., Caputi, P., & Oades, L. (2006). Stages of recovery instrument: Development of a measure of recovery from serious mental illness. *Australian & New Zealand Journal of Psychiatry, 40*(11), 972–980.

Andresen, R., Oades, L. G., & Caputi, P. (2003). The experience of recovery from schizophrenia: towards an empirically validated stage model. *Australian and New Zealand Journal of Psychiatry, 37*(5), 586–594.

Arbuthnott, A. E., & Lewis, S. P. (2015). Parents of youth who self-injure: A review of the literature and implications for mental health professionals. *Child and Adolescent Psychiatry and Mental Health, 9*(1), 35.

Baetens, I., Claes, L., Martin, G., Onghena, P., Grietens, H., Van Leeuwen, K., . . . & Griffith, J. W. (2014). Is nonsuicidal self-injury associated with parenting and family factors?. *The Journal of Early Adolescence, 34*(3), 387–405.

Bresin, K., & Schoenleber, M. (2015). Gender differences in the prevalence of nonsuicidal self-injury: A meta-analysis. *Clinical Psychology Review, 38*, 55–64.

Boas, F. (2013). *The mind of primitive man.* BoD–Books on Demand.

Brown, M. Z., Comtois, C. A., & Linehan, M. M. (2002). Reasons for suicide attempts and nonsuicidal self-injury in women with borderline personality disorder. *Journal of Abnormal Psychology, 111*(1), 198–202.

Brumariu, L. E., & Kerns, K. A. (2010). Parent–child attachment and internalizing symptoms in childhood and adolescence: A review of empirical findings and future directions. *Development and Psychopathology, 22*(1), 177–203.

Brumberg, J. J. (1997). *The body project: An intimate history of American girls.* New York: Vintage.

Brumberg, J. J. (2006). Are we facing an epidemic of self-injury? *Chronicle of Higher Education, 53*(16), B6.

Burns, D. D. (1980). *Feeling good: The new mood therapy.* New York: William Morrow and Co.

Byrne, S., Morgan, S., Fitzpatrick, C., Boylan, C., Crowley, S., Gahan, H., . . . & Guerin, S. (2008). Deliberate self-harm in children and adolescents: A qualitative study exploring the needs of parents and carers. *Clinical Child Psychology and Psychiatry, 13*(4), 493–504. doi: 10.1177/1359104508096765;

Chapman, A. L., Gratz, K. L., & Brown, M. Z. (2006). Solving the puzzle of deliberate self-harm: The experiential avoidance model. *Behaviour Research and Therapy, 44*, 371–394.

Chiesa, A., & Serretti, A. (2010). A systematic review of neurobiological and clinical features of mindfulness meditations. *Psychological Medicine, 40*(8), 1239–1252.

Cox, L. J., Stanley, B. H., Melhem, N. M., Oquendo, M. A., Birmaher, B., Burke, A., . . . & Brent, D. A. (2012). A longitudinal study of nonsuicidal self-injury in offspring at high risk for mood disorder. *Journal of Clinical Psychiatry, 73*(6), 821.

Diamond, G. S., Reis, B. F., Diamond, G. M., Siqueland, L., & Isaacs, L. (2002). Attachment-based family therapy for depressed adolescents: A treatment development study. *Journal of the American Academy of Child & Adolescent Psychiatry, 41*(10), 1190–1196.

Di Pierro, R., Sarno, I., Perego, S., Gallucci, M., & Madeddu, F. (2012). Adolescent nonsuicidal self-injury: The effects of personality traits, family relationships and maltreatment on the presence and severity of behaviours. *European Child & Adolescent Psychiatry, 21*(9), 511–520.

Duncan, L. G., Coatsworth, J. D., & Greenberg, M. T. (2009). A model of mindful parenting: Implications for parent–child relationships and prevention research. *Clinical Child and Family Psychology Review, 12*(3), 255–270.

Dweck, C. S. (2012). *Mindset: How you can fulfill your potential.* London: Constable & Robinson Limited.

D'Zurilla, T. J., & Nezu, A. M. (2001). Problem solving therapies. In K. Dobson (Ed.), *Handbook of cognitive-behavioral therapies* (2nd ed., pp. 211–245). New York: Guilford Press.

Esposito-Smythers, C., Spirito, A., Kahler, C. W., Hunt, J., & Monti, P. (2011). Treatment of co-occurring substance abuse and suicidality among adolescents: A randomized trial. *Journal of Consulting and Clinical Psychology, 79*(6), 728.

Evans, K., Tyrer, P., Catalan, J., Schmidt, U., Davidson, K., Dent, J., . . . & Thompson, S. (1999). Manual-assisted cognitive-behaviour therapy (MACT): A randomized controlled trial of a brief intervention with bibliotherapy in the treatment of recurrent deliberate self-harm. *Psychological Medicine, 29*(1), 19–25.

Favazza, A. R. (1996). *Bodies under siege: Self-mutilation and body modification in culture and psychiatry* (2nd ed.). Baltimore, MD: Johns Hopkins University Press.

Fleischhaker, C., Böhme, R., Sixt, B., Brück, C., Schneider, C., & Schulz, E. (2011). Dialectical behavioral therapy for adolescents (DBT-A): A clinical trial for patients with suicidal and self-injurious behavior and borderline symptoms with a one-year follow-up. *Child and Adolescent Psychiatry and Mental Health, 5*(1), 3.

Fox, K. R., Franklin, J. C., Ribeiro, J. D., Kleiman, E. M., Bentley, K. H., & Nock, M. K. (2015). Meta-analysis of risk factors for nonsuicidal self-injury. *Clinical Psychology Review, 42*, 156–167.

Franklin, J. C., Lee, K. M., Hanna, E. K., & Prinstein, M. J. (2013). Feeling worse to feel better: Pain-offset relief simultaneously stimulates positive affect and reduces negative affect. *Psychological Science, 24*(4), 521–529.

Garland, E. L., Fredrickson, B., Kring, A. M., Johnson, D. P., Meyer, P. S., & Penn, D. L. (2010). Upward spirals of positive emotions counter downward spirals of negativity: Insights from the broaden-and-build theory and affective neuroscience on the treatment of emotion dysfunctions and deficits in psychopathology. *Clinical Psychology Review, 30*(7), 849–864.

Gilbert, K. E. (2012). The neglected role of positive emotion in adolescent psychopathology. *Clinical Psychology Review, 32*(6), 467–467–481.

Gilbert, P. (1998). The evolved basis and adaptive functions of cognitive distortions. *Psychology and Psychotherapy: Theory, Research and Practice, 71*(4), 447–463.

Glassman, L. H., Weierich, M. R., Hooley, J. M., Deliberto, T. L., & Nock, M. K. (2007). Child maltreatment, non-suicidal self-injury, and the mediating role of self-criticism. *Behaviour Research and Therapy, 45*(10), 2483–2490.

Glenn, C. R., Franklin, J. C., & Nock, M. K. (2015). Evidence-based psychosocial treatments for self-injurious thoughts and behaviors in youth. *Journal of Clinical Child & Adolescent Psychology, 44*(1), 1–29.

Groschwitz, R. C., & Plener, P. L. (2012). The neurobiology of non-suicidal self-injury (NSSI). *Suicidology Online, 3,* 24–32.

Harper, G. P. (2012). Psychopharmacological Treatment. In B. W. Walsh (Ed.), *Treating self-injury: A practical guide* (2nd ed., pp. 195–203). New York: Guilford Press.

Hawton, K., Rodham, K., Evans, E., & Weatherall, R. (2002). Deliberate self harm in adolescents: Self report survey in schools in england. *British Medical Journal, 325,* 1207–1211

Hawton, K., Saunders, K. E. A., & O'Connor, R. C. (2012). Self-harm and suicide in adolescents. *Lancet, 379,* 2373–2382.

Healthypsych. (n. d.). What Is Family Therapy? Retrieved from https:// healthypsych.com/family-therapy/

Hilt, L. M., Nock, M. K., Lloyd-Richardson, E. E., & Prinstein, M. J. (2008). Longitudinal study of nonsuicidal self-injury among young adolescents: Rates, correlates, and preliminary test of an interpersonal model. *Journal of Early Adolescence, 28*(3), 455–469.

Hollander, M. (2008). *Helping teens who cut: Understanding and ending self-injury.* New York: Guilford Press.

Hollander, M. H. (2012). Family therapy. In B. W. Walsh (Ed.), *Treating self-injury: A practical guide* (2nd ed.). New York: Guilford Press.

Hyde, A. L., Conroy, D. E., Pincus, A. L., & Ram, N. (2011). Unpacking the feel-good effect of free-time physical activity: Between- and within-person associations with pleasant-activated feeling states. *Journal of Sport & Exercise Psychology, 33*, 884–902.

Jobes, D. A., Rudd, M. D., Overholser, J. C., & Joiner Jr, T. E. (2008). Ethical and competent care of suicidal patients: Contemporary challenges, new developments, and considerations for clinical practice. *Professional Psychology: Research and Practice, 39*(4), 405.

Josefsson, T., Lindwall, M., & Archer, T. (2014). Physical exercise intervention in depressive disorders: Meta-analysis and systematic review. *Scandinavian Journal of Medicine & Science in Sports, 24*, 259e272.

Kabat-Zinn, J. (2003). Mindfulness-based interventions in context: Past, present, and future. *Clinical Psychology: Science and Practice, 10*(2), 144–156.

Kabat-Zinn, M. (2009). *Everyday blessings: The inner work of mindful parenting.* New York, NY: Hatchette Book Group.

Kelada, L., Hasking, P., & Melvin, G. (2016). The relationship between nonsuicidal self-injury and family functioning: Adolescent and parent perspectives. *Journal of Marital and Family Therapy, 42*(3), 536–549.

Kelada, L., Whitlock, J., Hasking, P., & Melvin, G. (2016). Parents' experiences of nonsuicidal self-injury among adolescents and young adults. *Journal of Child and Family Studies, 25*(11), 3403–3416.

Kendall, P. C., Hudson, J. L., Gosch, E., Flannery-Schroeder, E., & Suveg, C. (2008). Cognitive-behavioral therapy for anxiety disordered youth: A randomized clinical trial evaluating child and family modalities. *Journal of Consulting and Clinical Psychology, 76*(2), 282–297.

Kleindienst, N., Bohus, M., Ludascher, P., Limberger, M. F., Kuenkele, K., Ebner-Priemer, U. W., Chapman, A. L., Reicherzer, M., Stieglitz, R. D., & Schmahl, C. (2008). Motives for nonsuicidal self-injury among women with borderline personality disorder. *Journal of Nervous and Mental Disorders, 196*(3), 230–236.

Klonsky, E. D. (2011). Nonsuicidal self-injury in United States adults: Prevalence, sociodemographics, topography and functions. *Psychological Medicine, 41*(9), 1981–1986.

Klonsky, E. D., & Glenn, C. R. (2008). Resisting urges to self-injure. *Behavioural and Cognitive Psychotherapy, 36*, 211–220.

Lader, W. (2006). A look at the increase in body focused behaviors. *Paradigm, 11*, 14–18.

Linehan, M. (1993). *Cognitive-behavioral treatment of borderline personality disorder.* New York: Guilford Press.

Linehan, M. (2014). *DBT skills training manual.* New York: Guilford Press.

Linehan, M. M., Heard, H. L., & Armstrong, H. E. (1993). Naturalistic follow-up of a behavioral treatment for chronically parasuicidal borderline patients. *Archives of General Psychiatry, 50*(12), 971–974.

Lloyd-Richardson, E. E., Perrine, N., Dierker, L., & Kelley, M. L. (2007). Characteristics of non-suicidal self-injury in a community sample of adolescents. *Psychological Medicine, 37*(8), 1183–1192.

Maciejewski, D. F., Creemers, H., Lynskey, M. T., Madden, P. A. F., Heath, A. C., Statham, D. J., . . . & Verweij, K. J. H. (2014). Different outcomes, same etiology? Shared genetic and environmental influences on non-suicidal self injury and suicidal ideation. *JAMA Psychiatry, 71*(6), 699–705.

Mangels, J. A., Butterfield, B., Lamb, J., Good, C., & Dweck, C. S. (2006). Why do beliefs about intelligence influence learning success? A social cognitive neuroscience model. *Social Cognitive and Affective Neuroscience, 1*(2), 75–86.

Marchant, A., Hawton, K., Stewart, A., Montgomery, P., Singaravelu, V., Lloyd, K., & John, A. (2017). A systematic review of the relationship between internet use, self-harm and suicidal behaviour in young people: The good, the bad and the unknown. *PLoS One, 12*(8), e0181722.

Marotz, L. R., & Kupzyk, S. (2018). *Parenting today's children: A developmental perspective.*Boston: Cengage Learning.

Martin, G., Swannell, S., Harrison, J., Hazell, P., & Taylor, A. (2010). *The Australian national epidemiological study of self-injury (ANESSI)* (No. 1, pp. 1–44). Queensland, AU: Centre for Suicide Prevention Studies

McGowan, P. O., Sasaki, A., D'alessio, A. C., Dymov, S., Labonté, B., Szyf, M., . . . & Meaney, M. J. (2009). Epigenetic regulation of the glucocorticoid receptor in human brain associates with childhood abuse. *Nature Neuroscience, 12*(3), 342–348.

McPhie, M. L., & Rawana, J. S. (2015). The effect of physical activity on depression in adolescence and emerging adulthood: A growth-curve analysis. *Journal of Adolescence*, 83–92.

Merikangas, K. R., He, J-P., Burstein, M., Swanson, S. A., Avenevoli, S., Cui, L., Benjet, C., et al. (2010). Lifetime prevalence of mental disorders in US adolescents: Results from the National Comorbidity Study—Adolescent Supplement (NCS-A). *Journal of the American Academy of Child and Adolescent Psychiatry, 49*(10), 980–989.

Muehlenkamp, J., Brausch, A., Quigley, B., & Whitlock, J. (2012). Interpersonal features and functions of NSSI. *Suicide and Life Threating Behavior, 43*(1): 67–80.

Muehlenkamp, J. J. (2006). Empirically supported treatments and general therapy guidelines for non-suicidal self-injury. *Journal of Mental Health Counseling, 28*(2), 166–185.

Muehlenkamp, J. J., Hilt, L. M., Ehlinger, P. P., & McMillan, T. (2015). Nonsuicidal self-injury in sexual minority college students: A test of theoretical integration. *Child and Adolescent Psychiatry and Mental Health, 9*(1), 16.

Nickel, M. K., Loew, T. H., & Gil, F. P. (2007). Aripiprazole in treatment of borderline patients, part II: An 18-month follow-up. *Psychopharmacology, 191*(4), 1023–1026.

Nickel, M. K., Muehlbacher, M., Nickel, C., Kettler, C., Gil, F. P., Bachler, E., . . . & Anvar, J. (2006). Aripiprazole in the treatment of patients with borderline personality disorder: A double-blind, placebo-controlled study. *American Journal of Psychiatry, 163*(5), 833–838.

Nock, M. K., Joiner, T. E., Gordon, K. H., Lloyd-Richardson, E., & Prinstein, M. J. (2007). Non-suicidal self-injury among adolescents: Diagnostic correlates and relation to suicide attempts. *Psychiatry Research, 144*(1), 65–72.

Nock, M. K., & Mendes, W. B. (2008). Physiological arousal, distress tolerance, and social problem-solving deficits among adolescent self-injurers. *Journal of Consulting and Clinical Psychology, 76*(1), 28

Oldershaw, A., Richards, C., Simic, M., & Schmidt, U. (2008). Parents' perspectives on adolescent self-harm: Qualitative study. *British Journal of Psychiatry, 193*(2), 140–144. doi: 10.1192/bjp.bp.107.045930;

Pietrusza, C., Rothenberg, P., & Whitlock, J. (2011, June). *Reaching out: The role of disclosure and support in non-suicidal self-injuruy.* Poster session presented at the 6th annual meeting of the International Society for the Study of Self-Injury (ISSS), New York.

Pineda, J., & Dadds, M. R. (2013). Family intervention for adolescents with suicidal behavior: A randomized controlled trial and mediation analysis. *Journal of the American Academy of Child & Adolescent Psychiatry, 52*(8), 851–862.

Plener, P. L., Libal, G., & Nixon, M. K. (2009). Use of medication in the treatment of nonsuicidal self-injury in youth. In M. K. Nixon & N. L. Heath (Eds.), *Self-injury in youth: The essential guide to assessment and intervention* (pp. 275–308). New York: Routledge/Taylor & Francis Group.

Prochaska, J. O., DiClemente, C. C., & Norcross, J. C. (1992). In search of the structure of change. In Y. Klar, J. D. Fisher, J. M. Chinsky, & A. Nadler (Eds.), *Self change* (pp. 87–114). New York: Springer.

Purington, A., Whitlock, J., & Pochtar, R. (2009). Non-suicidal self-injury in secondary schools: A descriptive study of prevalence, characteristics, and interventions. *Manuscript submitted for publication.*

Rathus, J. H., & Miller, A. L. (2002). Dialectical behavior therapy adapted for suicidal adolescents. *Suicide and Life-Threatening Behavior, 32*(2), 146–157.

Roepke, A. M., & Seligman, M. E. (2015). Doors opening: A mechanism for growth after adversity. *Journal of Positive Psychology, 10*(2), 107–115.

Ross, S., Heath, N. L., & Toste, J. R. (2009). Non-suicidal self-injury and eating pathology in high school students. *American Journal of Orthopsychiatry, 79*(1), 83–92.

Sandman, C. A. (2009). Psychopharmacologic treatment of nonsuicidal self-injury. In M. K. Nock (Ed.), *Understanding nonsuicidal self-injury: Origins, assessment, and treatment* (pp. 291–322). Washington, DC: American Psychological Association Press.

Serras, A., Saules, K. K., Cranford, J. A., & Eisenberg, D. (2010). Self-injury, substance use, and associated risk factors in a multi-campus probability sample of college students. *Psychology of Addictive Behaviors, 24*(1), 119–128.

Sher, L., & Stanley, B. (2009). Biological models of nonsuicidal self-injury. In M. K. Nock (Ed.), *Understanding nonsuicidal self-injury: Origins, assessment, and treatment.* Washington, DC: American Psychological Association Press.

Spirito, A., Esposito-Smythers, C., Wolff, J., & Uhl, E. (2011). History of cognitive-behavioral therapy in youth. *Child and Adolescent Psychiatric Clinics of North America, 20*(2), 179–189

Stanton, R., Happell, B., Hayman, M., & Reaburn, P. (2014). Exercise interventions for the treatment of affective disorders e research to practice. *Frontiers in Psychiatry, 5*, 46.

Steinberg, L., & Morris, A. S. (2001). Adolescent development. *Annual Review of Psychology, 52*(1), 83–110.

Swannell, S. V., Martin, G. E., Page, A., Hasking, P., & St John, N. J. (2014). Prevalence of nonsuicidal self-injury in nonclinical samples: Systematic review, meta-analysis and meta-regression. *Suicide and Life-Threatening Behavior, 44*(3), 273–303.

Thayer, R. E., Newman, J. R., & McClain, T. M. (1994). Self-regulation of mood: Strategies for changing a bad mood, raising energy, and reducing tension. *Journal of Personality and Social Psychology, 67*(5), 910–925.

Townsend, E., Hawton, K., Altman, D. G., Arensman, E., Gunnell, D., Hazell, P., . . . & Van Heeringen, K. (2001). The efficacy of problem-solving treatments after deliberate self-harm: Meta-analysis of randomized controlled trials with respect to depression, hopelessness and improvement in problems. *Psychological Medicine, 31*(6), 979–988.

Turner, B. J., Austin, S. B., & Chapman, A. L. (2015). Treating nonsuicidal self-injury: A systematic review of psychological and pharmacological interventions. *Canadian Journal of Psychiatry, 59*(11), 576–585.

Tyrer, P., Thompson, S., Schmidt, U., Jones, V., Knapp, M., Davidson, K., . . . & Byrne, G. (2003). Randomized controlled trial of brief cognitive behaviour therapy versus treatment as usual in recurrent deliberate self-harm: The POPMACT study. *Psychological Medicine, 33*(6), 969–976.

US Department of Health and Human Services. (2008). 2008 Physical Activity Guidelines for American. https://health.gov/paguidelines/pdf/paguide.pdf

Victor, S. E., & Klonsky, E. D. (2014a). Correlates of suicide attempts among self-injurers: A meta-analysis. *Clinical Psychology Review, 34*(4), 282–297. doi:10.1016/j.cpr.2014.03.005

Victor, S. E., & Klonsky, E. D. (2014b). Daily emotion in non-suicidal self-injury. *Journal of Clinical Psychology, 70*(4), 364–375.

Wallenstein, M. B., & Nock, M. K. (2007). Physical exercise as a treatment for non-suicidal self-injury: Evidence from a single-case study. *American Journal of Psychiatry, 164*(2), 350–351.

Walsh, B. W. (2012). *Treating self-injury: A practical guide* (2nd ed.). New York: Guilford Press.

Weaver, I. C., Cervoni, N., Champagne, F. A., D'Alessio, A. C., Sharma, S., Seckl, J. R., . . . & Meaney, M. J. (2004). Epigenetic programming by maternal behavior. *Nature Neuroscience, 7*(8), 847–854.

Wedig, M. M., & Nock, M. K. (2007). Expressed emotion and adolescent self-injury. *Journal of the American Academy of Child & Adolescent Psychiatry, 46*(9), 1171–1178.

Whitlock, J., Lloyd-Richardson, E., Fisseha, F., & Bates, T. (2017). Parental secondary stress: The often hidden but important underbelly of non-suicidal self-injury in youth. *Journal of Clinical Psychology*: doi:10.1002/jclp.22488

Whitlock, J., Muehlenkamp, J., Eckenrode, J., Purington, A., Barrera, P., Baral-Abrams, G., . . . & Smith, E. (2013). Non-suicidal self-injury as a gateway to suicide in adolescents and young adults. *Journal of Adolescent Health, 52*(4): 486–492.

Whitlock, J., Muehlenkamp, J., Purington, A., Eckenrode, J., Barreira, J., Abrams, . . . & Knox, K. (2011). Non-suicidal self-injury in a college population: General trends and sex differences. *Journal of American College Health, 59*(8): 691–698.

Whitlock, J. L., Prussein, K., & Pietrusza, C. (2015). Predictors of non-suicidal self-injury and psychological growth. *Child and Adolescent Psychiatry and Mental Health, 9*(19). doi: 10.1186/s13034-015-0048-5. PMCID: PMC4495705

Whitlock, J. L., Purington, A., & Gershkovich, M. (2009). Influence of the media on self-injurious behavior. In M. Nock (Ed.), *Understanding non-suicidal self-injury current science and practice* (pp. 139–156). Washington, DC: American Psychological Association Press.

Whitlock, J. L., & Selekman, M. (2014). Non-suicidal self-injury (NSSI) across the lifespan. In M. Nock (Ed.), *Oxford handbook of suicide and self-injury* (pp. 133–154). New York, NY: Oxford Library of Psychology, Oxford University Press.

Wood, A. M., Froh, J. J., & Geraghty, A. W. (2010). Gratitude and well-being: A review and theoretical integration. *Clinical Psychology Review, 30*(7), 890–905.

Yehuda, R., & Bierer, L. M. (2007). Transgenerational transmission of cortisol and PTSD risk. *Progress in Brain Research, 167,* 121–135

Zeanah, C. H., Smyke, A. T., Koga, S. F., Carlson, E., & The Bucharest Early Intervention Project Core Group. (2005). Attachment in institutionalized and community children in Romania. *Child Development, 76*(5), 1015–1028.

Zetterqvist, M. (2015). The DSM-5 diagnosis of nonsuicidal self-injury disorder: A review of the empirical literature. *Child and Adolescent Psychiatry and Mental Health.* https://doi.org/10.1186/s13034-015-0062-7

About the Authors

Janis Whitlock, PhD, is a research scientist in the Bronfenbrenner Center for Translational Research at Cornell University and the founder and director of the Cornell Research Program on Self-Injury and Recovery. Dedicated to linking cutting-edge science with on-the-ground efforts to support and enhance the lives of youth and their families, her research focuses on adolescent and young adult social and emotional health and well-being, sexual violence prevention, and the role of social media in health and development. She is best known for her work on nonsuicidal self-injury. In addition to conducting research in these areas, she is dedicated to making research accessible and useful to those best positioned to make a difference in the lives of youth, such as parents and youth-serving professionals.

Elizabeth Lloyd-Richardson, PhD, is an associate professor of psychology at the University of Massachusetts Dartmouth. She is a licensed clinical psychologist with specialized training in adolescent health risk behaviors. She began conducting research on and interviewing teens who self-injure nearly two decades ago and has extensive experience in developing and running research programs that aim to promote healthful behaviors in adolescents and young adults. She has authored more than 60 papers and book chapters in the areas of nonsuicidal self-injury, weight management, and substance use and abuse.

Index